T0385315

How the Art of Medicine Makes the Science More Effective

BECOMING THE MEDICINE WE PRACTICE

Dr. Claudia Welch, DOM
Foreword by Dr. Robert Svoboda, BAMS

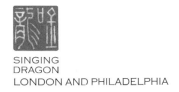

SINGING
DRAGON
LONDON AND PHILADELPHIA

First published in 2015
by Singing Dragon
an imprint of Jessica Kingsley Publishers
73 Collier Street
London N1 9BE, UK
and
400 Market Street, Suite 400
Philadelphia, PA 19106, USA

www.singingdragon.com

Library of Congress Cataloging in Publication Data
Welch, Claudia, author.
  How the art of medicine makes the science more effective : becoming the medicine we practice / Claudia Welch.
    p. ; cm.
  Includes bibliographical references.
  ISBN 978-1-84819-229-4 (alk. paper)
  I. Title.
  [DNLM: 1. Attitude of Health Personnel. 2. Physicians--standards. 3. Clinical Competence. 4. Physician's Role. 5. Physician-Patient Relations. W 62]
  R690
  610.69--dc23

                        2015014572

British Library Cataloguing in Publication Data
A CIP catalogue record for this book is available from the British Library

ISBN 978 1 84819 229 4
eISBN 978 0 85701 181 7

Printed and bound in the United States

Dedicated to the Effective Physician

CONTENTS

Foreword

For a doctor, a patient is a book open to a page that requires reading and interpretation. Each human "book" is a singular story, written by that individual and his or her enveloping environment, a tale of choices made and experiences undergone that have developed into illness and must now be edited and revised, that it may lead into health. The challenge of medicine is that each book is written in its own idiosyncratic language that is only partly discernible by the rational mind.

For all the knowledge it can offer us about diseases and therapies, science cannot provide us with the specifics needed to address the singularity of the person sitting in front of us; medicine comes alive and works through us only when it becomes elevated from science into art. Doctors become medicine when their inner and outer realities become well-oriented with the life force so that that life force may flow through them to do the work of healing.

Though none of us may ever attain the level of alignment reached by that Great Physician who radiated such curative power that one could be healed simply by touching the hem of His garment, each of us who has taken the vow to serve life by serving the living as a physician can honor that life by assisting the life force to flow better through those living bodies. In doing so, we ourselves receive the boon of the healing we have striven to embody.

Fate has rendered me perhaps uniquely qualified to bear witness to the path that the author of this book has followed as she has worked to become the medicine she practices. Though I first met

Dr. Claudia Welch in the mid-eighties when she was still a teen, our acquaintance blossomed during the year she spent at age 20 studying Hindi (and surviving India) in Varanasi. That was nearly 30 years ago, and in the ensuing decades I've known her first as a dedicated student, then as a valued colleague, and always as a dear and trusted friend. Many and varied are the experiences we've shared, including particularly the experience of teaching together, in 12 different countries thus far. Having thus enjoyed the opportunity to participate in her development both as a professional and as a human being, I can testify to Dr. Welch's dedication and sincerity, her reliability, and her determination always to offer her best. Moreover, not only has every patient that I have referred to her reported (sometimes astonishing) benefit, I have on more than one occasion myself profited by her treatment.

As a sincere disciple she strives hard to follow her guru's precepts, in particular his instruction that a physician should always think she can find the cure for the pain of the patient, and when she can offer nothing else, to at least offer compassion. This new book of hers is a vade mecum for all healers who wish to themselves embody healing compassion and become the medicine that they practice.

Robert Svoboda, Ayurvedacharya
Costa Rica, 2015

ACKNOWLEDGMENTS

Obeisance be to that unparalleled Physician who has
completely destroyed diseases like passion or desire, etc.[1]
which are constantly associated with and spread all over the
body, giving rise to anxiety, delusion and restlessness.
VAGBHATTA[2]

My spiritual teachers and lineage. For sharing their expertise, experience, and inspiration in many and varied ways over time—sometimes a lot of time: Dr. Jim Ventresca, Dr. Robert E. Svoboda, Dr. Vasant Lad, Jessica Kingsley, Margot Silk Forrest, Fred Smith, Ph.D., Durga Leela, B.A., Russell Perkins, MTS, Om Prakash Sharma ji (RIP), Dr. Chuck Ventresca, Dr. Yimen Xu, Ray Lowe, M.A., Pamela Kentish, L.Ac., Edward Kentish, L.Ac., Dr. Eduardo Cardona-Sanclemente, Dr. Larry Dossey, Rick Silberman, and Beecher Grogan. For letting me take up space and keeping me company—or quiet—while I wrote: Jon and Ann Sairs, J. R. R. Franklin, Sarah Lowther, and the staff at Shipwreck Café. For their stories and conversations about medicine: Sam Colt, Greta Lowther, Eric Perkins, Dr. Peter Wong, M.D., Thomas Hughes, L.Ac., and my friends and patients—both the lucky and the unlucky ones. For all their efforts, conscious or otherwise: healthcare practitioners, and anyone else who strives in their own ways to become medicine.

PREFACE AND NOTES

The fish trap exists because of the fish. Once you've gotten the fish,
you can forget the trap. The rabbit snare exists because of the rabbit.
Once you've gotten the rabbit, you can forget the snare.
Words exist because of meaning. Once you've gotten the meaning,
you can forget the words. Where can I find a man who
has forgotten the words so I can talk with him?
CHUANG TZU[1]

This quote expresses the challenge for me in writing this book. It is so easy to offend without intending to. I request tolerance as we work together to look beyond the words, to share in the spirit of exploration and communication. Just as it can be subjective or difficult to describe what makes a work of fine art excellent, so too with the art of medicine.

Given the many physicians who have been active in their medical practices for longer than I—and with more insight and experience— it seems almost presumptuous to write about the art of medicine. Had I not been asked by publisher Jessica Kingsley to write a book on this topic, I probably would not have chosen to. But when asked, especially by such a thoughtful woman, I recalled Ben Franklin, who is said to have made it a habit not to seek out positions or obligations, but to try to accept them when they landed in his lap. So I agreed to explore the elements, insights, and sometimes difficult personal experiences of this art, both as a student of medicine and human nature, and having worked as a healthcare practitioner.

Much has been written on the doctor–patient relationship in the Western scientific canon. While I do take some of these studies into consideration in this book, I mostly rely on Eastern thought— especially Ayurveda—to guide this exploration. I have made an effort to include important passages from Ayurvedic texts that pertain to the subjects in this book, as well as directives from my guru to me, in order to ground this discussion in true authority. More about authority later.

For areas in which I have less experience, I have turned to the counsel and experience of practitioners with more extensive training and background. God willing, the insights and explorations in these pages will resonate with and support good medicine, or trigger conversations or insights of equal or greater value.

While I organize this book around the four qualities ancient Ayurveda considered prerequisites to be an effective physician, I think the information and explorations in these pages could serve practitioners and physicians from any medical tradition. In fact, because this book is in great measure about relationships, I find many of the skills explored here useful in day-to-day interactions outside a medical practice, so I think anyone might find it useful. With this in mind, whenever I use the word "doctor" or "physician," I really mean anybody who is practicing healthcare, from physicians to nurses, counselors, massage therapists, psychologists, yoga therapists, to parents. And when I talk about prescriptions, I mean everything from antibiotics, to lifestyle recommendations.

When discussing any art it is easy to sound, or become, divorced from practicality, untethered to reality. Whether trying to describe a work of Picasso or how a patient and doctor communicate, it is a challenge to keep such a decidedly real experience *real*, rather than vague, abstract, New-Agey, or irritating. For example, in some of the best moments of medicine, it can feel to both the doctor and the patient that something profound is going on. How do we break that down into components to examine? How do we cultivate it? How do we learn, teach, explain, or even talk about it? We may want to connect in the most healing and helpful way possible with our patients, but to talk about it…well, that can feel gauche.

In navigating these challenges, and others inherent in exploring the topics in this book, I apologize for any instance where I fall short or am mistaken, misguided, or just downright wrong. It is bound to happen.

A Few Notes Before We Begin

- When I do not capitalize organ names, like liver, I am referring to them in the context of Western physiology. If I do capitalize them, like Liver, I am referring to them in the context of Eastern medicine. The understanding of the organs is a bit different in the different medical traditions.

- All the names and particulars in the case studies here have been altered to protect privacy, but in such a manner as to retain the spirit of the stories. The story of Sam Colt is an exception. She preferred that I include her name and the particulars of her story.

- I use the words and concepts of God, Good Orderly Direction (G.O.D.), Divinity, Real, and Good fairly interchangeably. If you wonder about the presence of any one of these energies or entities, I don't think my beliefs will be an obstructive influence in this book.

- At the beginning of many chapters, I include quotes; sometimes quite a few. Sometimes these are dense and archaic. I have chosen to include them anyway, as they relate to ideas in the chapters they introduce, and some medical students and practitioners are—and this may be hard to believe with some of these quotes—delighted by reading the original references. Also, I like the authority they add. If you are not delighted by them, however, there is no harm in skipping them.

- Part I is dense. Hang in there, or skip ahead if you're not in the mood. It gets easier after that. Chapter 1 is not only dense, but it refers more to Western medical issues than the rest of the book. Again, if you're not in the mood, no problem with skipping a bit. In fact, there is no harm in skipping around in general.

- For the Sanskrit terms in this book, I am choosing to sacrifice standard transliteration rules, to use the most common spellings that will encourage the most accurate pronunciation from the majority of readers.

Introduction
The Art of Medicine and the Four Qualities of a Physician

A physician, well versed in the principles of the theory of medicine, but unskilful in his art through want of practice, loses his wit at the bedside of his patient, just as a coward is panicked and at a loss to determine what to do when for the first time he finds himself in the ranks of a contending army. On the other hand, a physician experienced in his art but lacking in the theory of medicine, is condemned by all good men as a quack and deserves capital punishment at the hands of the king. Both these classes of physicians are untrustworthy because they are half educated. Such men are as capable of discharging their duties just as a one-winged bird is capable of flight.
SUSHRUTA[1]

Excellence in theoretical knowledge, extensive practical experience, dexterity and purity—this is the quadruple of qualities of a physician.
CHARAKA[2]

In the modern-day version of the Hippocratic Oath, we vow to "remember that there is art to medicine as well as science, and that warmth, sympathy, and understanding may outweigh the surgeon's knife or the chemist's drug."

Weighty words indeed: "warmth, sympathy, and understanding may outweigh the surgeon's knife or the chemist's drug." While today's healthcare practitioners are schooled in the science of a chosen medical modality, we may falter when it comes to confidence in practicing the art of our craft.

There is no substitute for being well trained in a medical system. Having intuition and art to the exclusion of considerable study is like having hot air without the balloon. There can be no flight. Similarly, even a well-designed and excellently crafted balloon will remain limp without hot air to lift it. Both science and art are necessary to the effective practice of medicine. This book focuses on the art, presupposing the doctor has training in medical science. I have come to think of the main difference between the two as this: *In the science of medicine, we learn to dispense medicine. In the art, we learn to become it.*

Both the original and modern versions of the Hippocratic Oath have strong correlations with precepts given in ancient Eastern medicine classics, and Ayurvedic classical texts offer an especially elegant structure through which to explore the art of medicine.

Charaka, the author of *Charaka Samhita*, one of the preeminent, classic ancient Ayurvedic texts,[3] states that to achieve efficacy in medicine, four components or "legs" are required: a physician, a nurse, medicine, and a patient.[4] Because the last three are dependent on the counsel and direction of the physician, the physician is the most critical of the four, and should therefore strive to fill that role to the best of her ability.[5]

For the physician to be competent, Charaka tells us, he must possess four qualities: excellence in theoretical knowledge, extensive practical experience, dexterity, and purity.[6] The first four parts of this book are dedicated to the art associated with each of these qualities. The fifth part addresses the medicine component, since the responsibility of prescribing is that of the physician. The sixth part is just for fun.

For the purposes in this book, let us consider what each of these qualities contributes to the art of medicine—to our ability to become the medicine we practice.

PART I

Excellence in Theoretical Knowledge[1]

How We Know What We Know

That extremely severe disorders vanish like the (imaginary) city of gandharvas [musical spirits] and even simplest disorders aggravate in want of quick management in spite of the presence of the three other legs [the nurse, the medicine, and the patient], confirms that the learned and the ignorant physicians are responsible for the above two consequences respectively. (14)

It is better to self-immolate than to be treated by a physician ignorant of the science of medicine. As a blind man moves about with the help of the movement of his hands...so the ignorant physician proceeds in therapeutic management with too much trepidation. (15–16)

Such one regarding himself as physician, cures by accident a diseased person whose life-span is certain but, on the other hand, kills hundreds having uncertain life-span. (17)

Scriptures are like light for illumination and one's own intellect is like the eye. If endowed with both, the physician does not commit mistakes. Because in treatment, the (other) three legs are dependent on the physician, the physician should make all efforts to refine his own qualities. (24–25)
CHARAKA[2]

Excellence in theoretical knowledge is the first of the four qualities Charaka prescribes as necessary in order to be an effective physician. Over the course of Part I, let us consider how the pursuit of knowledge contributes to the art of medicine.

How do we know what we know? How do we know that what we do or prescribe for our patients is correct? Why do we know one treatment will be more effective than another, or that another would actually be harmful?

Let us explore this. Charaka tells us there are three valid sources of knowledge: authority, perception, and inference.[3] Let us look at the meaning of each of these, how we use them in the modern world, the shortcomings of relying on them too heavily, and how we might mine each of them for the best it has to offer.

1

Authority

Questioning Our Sources of Knowledge

What Constitutes Authority?

*Authority is the statement of the credible persons (apta).
Aptas are those who possess knowledge devoid of any doubt,
indirect or partial acquisition, attachment, or aversion. The
statement of such a person is valid testimony. On the contrary,
the statement of a drunkard, insane person, fool, or one who
is attached should not be considered valid testimony.*
CHARAKA[1]

*Now the definition of authority: those who are free from rajas and
tamas[2] and endowed with strength of penance and knowledge, and
whose knowledge is without defects, never contradicted, and true
universally in past, present, and future, are known as apta (who
have acquired all the knowledge), are expert in the discipline,
and enlightened; their word is free from doubt and is true because,
being devoid of rajas and tamas, how can they speak a lie?*
CHARAKA[3]

*The wise person who wishes to be a physician should first of all
examine the treatise with reason, keeping in consideration his
seriousness or otherwise in the work, result, after-effects, place,
and time. Various treatises on medicine are found in society, from
amongst them one should select that which is great, used by eminent*

and wise men, full of ideas, respected by authorities, intelligible, and beneficial to all the three types of disciples (dull, mediocre, and intelligent), free from the defect of repetition, coming down from the sages, with well-composed introduction, discussion, and conclusion, having firm base, free from weak and difficult words, having abundant expressions, with traditional ideas, devoted mainly to arriving at the essence of ideas, having consistent ideas, with demarcated topics, easily comprehensible, and having definitions illustrated with examples. Such treatise, like the clear sun illumines the entire subject while dispelling the darkness (of ignorance).
CHARAKA[4]

To practice medicine, we first need to learn it from an authoritative source. Who or what is worthy to be called an "authority"? Not many or much, it turns out.

According to Charaka, reliable authority is someone who is free from excessive mental or physical activity or stimulation, free from slothful, inert, hedonistic tendencies, and who is not attached to a particular outcome. Furthermore, she must be expert in her discipline and spiritually enlightened, and her knowledge must be universally true in past, present, and future.

Clearly, if this is true, most of us may be hard pressed to find even one living authority to which to turn for knowledge. If we are not so lucky to find a living authority, we may turn instead to other sources, including authoritative texts, our patients and Western scientific studies.

Authoritative Texts

The *Vedas*—a body of authoritative classical texts in India—are understood to be have been written by sages that fit Charaka's description of authority, so the texts themselves were traditionally considered authoritative, as were other ancient classics in Eastern medicine—in Ayurveda and Traditional Chinese Medicine (TCM), and the ancient classics of their sister sciences: Daoism, Feng Shui, Yoga, Tantra, Jyotisha, Sanskrit, Dance, Vastu Shastra, and tomes the world over written by enlightened beings.

When we study these various sister sciences and luminaries, we acquaint ourselves with authority. Our intellects sharpen as we learn the laws of nature and how they apply to human beings, and our hearts soften as we are influenced by the wisdom of the authors. When we explore the meaning and qualities of various aspects of our environment, we gain more understanding of the context and expression of life. If we are familiar with the context in which we and our patients live our lives, we can work with that environment to create more harmony within our environments.

There are shortcomings, however, when we take these ancient texts out of the context in which they were written. Very often they were written as a supplement to a predominantly oral tradition of medical knowledge and wisdom that was traditionally passed, in person, from teacher to student. If we take these texts as gospel rather than direction and inspiration, we might find ourselves neglecting one of the other three critical qualities of an effective physician: dexterity. We need to be flexible enough to apply the spirit and words of ancient sources, to the situations and unique complexities of the modern day, lest the doctor become a narrow-minded pulpiter and medicine become a dogmatic religion.

In our quest for knowledge, we may turn also to more modern texts, teachers and authors to find inspiration and education. But these may fall well short of Charaka's ambitious requirements for authority, so we would want to remember that there may be limitations, biases, or blatantly false information present in these sources of information. Even if the information is convincing. History has taught that today's consensus regularly becomes tomorrow's disproved folly. We will consider examples presently.

Our Patients

Another possible source of credible testimony may be patients themselves, provided they possess knowledge "devoid of any doubt, indirect and partial acquisition, attachment, and aversion," according to Charaka. Some patients may fit this description, as they know their own condition fully and directly, and are able to present it objectively.

On the contrary, says Charaka, when patients are addicted to harmful substances, mentally disturbed, or too "attached," their testimony should not be accepted as valid.[5] Though Charaka doesn't elaborate on what he means by "attached," we know that when someone is attached to a particular point of view or outcome, it influences her perceptions, just as attachment to a certain point of view or belief may bias research or perceptions of authors, professors, or doctors. More about that later.

So we can sometimes acquire limited knowledge from our patients—knowledge about their conditions—and we can acquire knowledge from ancient and modern textbooks, scriptures, and other inspired material, and from professors or teachers who come as close as possible to Charaka's ideal.

Once we leave school and become established in our medical practices, we may feel insecure about our knowledge—or lack thereof. It is not uncommon to begin to doubt the value of these authoritative sources, and to cast about for further confirmation from other authoritative sources. In the modern world, we often turn to Western scientific studies to gain more knowledge and confidence in our medicine, and to impart that knowledge to our patients.

I have seen this practice to be so widespread that I believe it is worthy of careful consideration.

Western Scientific Studies

We seem to have a global consensus that studies are, if not *the* way, at least a very good way to establish knowledge. In the US alone, we sink about US$100 billion a year into research,[6] and this research extends beyond Western medical drugs and treatments, to dietary factors and herbs from all traditions—Western, TCM, Ayurvedic, Tibetan, and others. Sometimes Complementary and Alternative Medical (CAM) practitioners feel that Western medicine is more advanced or prestigious, and we turn to its methods to validate our own.

Even if we don't consider Western medicine to be superior, we may lack confidence and seek to find it by placing our faith in studies. We may turn to Western scientific studies—or create our own based on the Western scientific method—to prove the efficacy of a therapy, herb, or medical approach we choose to use.

When we see positive results from a study on a particular therapy, herb, or medical approach, there are a few common reactions:

- We gain confidence in that medicine or therapy.

- We base our medical protocol or treatment strategy on the results and recommendations associated with those studies.

- We cite the study to our patients to instill confidence in them.

While we may think of the scientific process as objective, rigorous, and assiduous in assessing the truth, the reality is that the scientific process is vulnerable to a multitude of distorting influences that lead to faulty study design, execution, results, and result interpretation.

The number of sound, replicable studies is small, and nobody has done more to discover this than meta-researcher Dr. John Ioannidis, an epidemiologist at Stanford University, and one of the world's foremost experts on the credibility of modern medical research.

In one extensive study (yes, I recognize the irony of studying studies), Dr. Ioannidis found that out of 432 claims of *replicable* results, only a single study was consistently replicable. These studies were not necessarily poorly designed, either. Dr. Ioannidis found high levels of contradiction even in "gold standard" randomized controlled trials.[7]

In 2005, the *Journal of the American Medical Association* (*JAMA*) published a study by Dr. Ioannidis demonstrating that of the 49 medical studies most frequently cited in the 13 years leading up to his own study, *41 percent had been proven to be significantly exaggerated or wrong.*[8] This litany of troubles spawned books like *How to Lie With Statistics*, by Darrell Huff, even way back in 1993. It's not news, but we persist in treating statistics with reverence rather than caution.

The big problem with this, of course, is that we, as a medical community, use the results of these very often flawed studies as the basis for our medical protocols, prescriptive practices, treatment plans, surgery, and dietary and lifestyle advice. And we continue to do so even after a study's conclusions have been conclusively proven false.

Dr. Ioannidis charges that as much as 90 percent of the medical information directing medical protocol is flawed. He says 80 percent of the most common type of study—that is, non-randomized studies—are simply wrong, as are 25 percent of randomized trials—the so-called gold standard studies—and as much as 10 percent of the large randomized trials, or "platinum standard" studies.[9]

Why are so many of these studies flawed? Let us look at some of the problems involved.

Replicability

The test of replicability is considered the foundation of modern research. In theory, treatment protocols in Western medicine are "evidence-based." That is, we base our protocols and treatment strategies on the results of solid studies with replicable results. We assume that studies will be replicable and replicated, and their results will be stable. This is not always the case. It is, perhaps, rarely the case.

We are, for example, sometimes not even able to ensure replicability when studying something as foundational as the law of gravity. In one test, physicists used deep holes in the Nevada desert to measure gravity, and found a 2.5 percent discrepancy between the theoretical predictions and the data measured.[10]

Scientists, it turns out, have very little incentive to dedicate their time, energy, and resources to replicating other studies. One major disincentive is sheer cost. Another is that studies designed to replicate other studies are simply not likely to get published—and publication is a distinction of great value to researchers and research professors.

A Flair for the Dramatic

To achieve credibility, get funding for their next study, win tenured positions in universities, or even keep their jobs, researchers are often under relentless pressure to publish their work in reputable journals.

These reputable journals can have rejection rates of over 90 percent. The studies they do publish are likely to be ones with seemingly dramatic results. There is also a publication bias for positive results over negative results—negative findings are half as likely to be published as positive ones.[11]

Suppose a study is published that concludes a certain therapy is no more efficacious than a placebo. Now suppose that we have 15 studies that support this conclusion. Those are not exciting results. But if we have one study that refutes the conclusions of the initial study and finds the therapy efficacious, this is news. And it is more likely to get published than the 15 that replicated the original conclusion that the therapy was not efficacious. We may never even see those studies. They may not be published anywhere.

As conscientious physicians, we may read all the studies we can find about this therapy. If all we have access to is one study supporting and one study refuting its efficacy, we are likely to arrive at a very different conclusion than if we saw that, of 17 studies done, only one showed positive results.

In order to find a study likely to both meet significance-testing standards and have dramatic enough findings to be published, researchers have plenty of incentive to design studies that are likely to be dramatic, even if not wholly reflective of truth.

Peer Review vs. Peer Pressure

In the Western scientific community, we are supposed to carefully review, test, and replicate each other's work. This is supposed to be one of the main tools to protect against research error and bias, but it takes time, energy, and money that few researchers may possess, even if they have a desire to contribute to the pool of replicable studies.

While in theory the peer review process is supposed to keep the scientific field self-regulated and honest, we can also use it to suppress opposing opinions. Journals, for example, ask researchers to help them decide which studies to publish, and if those researchers disagree with outcomes in certain studies, they may be unlikely to recommend publication.[12]

Researchers themselves admit that faulty, biased, and even fraudulent studies are regularly published. In 2006, *Nature*, a reputable science journal, published an editorial that stated, "Scientists understand that peer review per se provides only a minimal assurance of quality, and that the public conception of peer review as a stamp of authentication is far from the truth."[13]

Bogus Scientific Journals

To add to the mess, there is also the growing phenomenon of bogus scientific journals. These may have very similar names to those of legitimate journals, but have nowhere near the same standards.

It is difficult for anyone but experienced researchers and readers to distinguish between credible articles and journals, and bogus ones. And there are plenty of bogus ones. One research librarian at the University of Colorado in Denver estimates that in 2013 there were as many as 4000 bogus journals—about 25 percent of the total number of open-access journals.[14]

These journals have an incentive to exist: they charge a fee for their authors to publish articles with them, a fee they may not advertise or even inform the author about until after their work has been published.[15]

So if we are taking published studies or journals as authority, we may not be on as solid ground as we'd like to believe. There are, however, resources to help us determine whether or not a journal is well regarded. One such resource is: www.sci-phy.com/detecting-bogus-scientific-journals.

Significance Chasing

For the past century or so, "significance testing" has governed research. The principle of "significance testing" dictates that in order to be considered significant, results of a study must demonstrate a less than 5 percent chance of occurring by...er...chance. This rather arbitrary number may impel scientists to manipulate data analyses or play with numbers in an attempt to show results that will render their study meaningful in the eyes of the scientific community—and more likely to get published.[16]

Psychologist Uri Simonsohn of the University of Pennsylvania and his colleagues have popularized a term for the self-deception researchers engage in whereby, consciously or otherwise, they manipulate data and numbers or alter methods until they suggest significant results. The term "P-hacking" is synonymous with other such practices: data-dredging, snooping, fishing, double-dipping, and significance chasing.[17] The simple fact that there are so many terms for this practice is telling.

Significance chasing, along with publication bias and selective reporting of results, is thought to be an important factor in the "decline effect." This is a term coined to describe the odd phenomenon whereby a drug becomes less and less effective the more scientists try to replicate the initial findings on it. If scientists conducting the initial research were engaged in "significance chasing," it is possible that their results conformed to their biases.[18] So naturally, future attempts to replicate these results would be less successful.

When we chase significance to the point of creating—and publishing—an illusion, it can take a very long time for the scientific community to see through that illusion. It takes time to create parameters and to execute studies to test our colleagues' results, and it may take decades to unravel what seemed to be tightly woven, well-established results.[19]

Bias and Belief Blindness

In China, Japan, and Taiwan between 1966 and 1995—a span of 29 years—100 percent of the 47 clinical trials studies concluded that acupuncture was an effective therapy. In the same time period, in the US, Sweden and the UK, only 56 percent of twice as many clinical trials found any therapeutic effects from acupuncture.

The fact that we see such conflicting studies suggests that researchers can find ways to confirm their biases, consciously or unconsciously. Our beliefs, if they do not blind us, may at least cause us to ask questions in such a way as to arrive at answers we like.[20] In this case, our results may be accurate, but the very questions that directed the study reflected a bias. Our beliefs may lead us to design, execute, or interpret a study in such a way that it is likely to shore up our biases.

Biases can simply reflect a preferred worldview, or they can be motivated by financial gain. One of the important questions to ask of any study is, "Who benefits from the results?" Particularly, "Who benefits financially?" If I am selling a product and I myself design, execute, and interpret a study to test that product's worthiness, I have a financial conflict of interest.

Here are some ways bias may shape research or results, both during the study and after it is completed.

- We can design a study on the effectiveness of a substance or therapy, comparing it to another substance or therapy already proven to be ineffective (or even harmful). Then, when our product or therapy proves more effective—or at least less harmful—than what we compared it to, we can claim it's superior. (It's like that old joke: you and your friend are running from a bear. To survive, you don't have to outrun the bear—you just have to outrun your buddy.) In order to claim superiority of a product, you simply prove it is less harmful than the other product.

- While the results of a study may show an improvement in patients' health after using a particular drug or therapy, it often fails to demonstrate that the drug or therapy was responsible for this change—or that the improvement was significant.

- Companies can focus research on subjective outcomes, like self-reported improvement ("I think my headache was better today"), rather than objective outcomes, like survival versus death. For example, a certain drug may provide subjective benefits like, "I think it helped my headache," but neglect the fact that the mortality rate is higher for patients who take it.

Financial Incentive

Studies, especially large ones, can be hugely expensive to conduct, and the money to conduct them has to come from somewhere. The group or business funding the research can, unfortunately, influence its outcome.[21] Not surprisingly, evidence suggests that when for-profit organizations study their products or services, they are more likely to find positive results than studies funded by not-for-profit organizations.[22] This suggests that, when there is no clear financial beneficiary of the studies' results, they may be more trustworthy.

Another question to ask is this: "Is the substance being studied patented or naturally occurring?" At the time of writing, it is not legal to patent a "product of nature," that is, a naturally occurring substance.[23] When a company patents something, they have exclusive right to sell it, so if a study "proves" the substance beneficial, the company could reap enormous financial benefit. This is a monumental financial prospect that does not apply to naturally occurring substances. If, for example, a study found that dandelions were very effective in the treatment of acne, we could all just pick them from our gardens. Whoever sponsored that study would not be able to recoup their investment by being the exclusive provider of dandelions. So there is far less financial incentive in general in studies of naturally occurring substances.

With this in mind, while I have not done or seen a platinum-standard meta-analysis to prove this, it seems quite possible that studies on naturally occurring substances have less bias, and are therefore more trustworthy. This may be good news for practitioners of medicines who rely on naturally occurring substances. Like herbs.

Reversals and Contradictions

Here is a very partial list of research findings and the reversals or contradictions the Western medical community has embraced in the last 20 years or so. These may have come about because of discovery of bias or poor research protocol in the original study, failed attempts to replicate previous studies, or conclusive disproof of the efficacy of once-standard drugs or practices.

Depending on which study or "authority" we consult we find that:

- Mammograms are an effective tool to detect cancer and save lives, *or* mammograms are not more effective, overall, in saving lives, and they cause more harm than benefit through the alarming false-positive readings they can produce.

- Colonoscopies and prostate-specific antigen (PSA) screenings are extremely important tools for cancer detection and need to be done frequently, *or* they shouldn't be done frequently because they do not necessarily save lives.

- Antidepressants such as Prozac, Zoloft, and Paxil, are effective medications, *or* they are no more effective than a placebo for most cases of depression.

- Cell phones cause brain cancer, *or* cell phones do not cause brain cancer.

- Exposure to the sun causes skin cancer, *or* avoiding direct sunlight entirely can increase risk of cancer.

- Sleeping more than eight hours a night is healthful, *or* it is dangerous to your health.

- Taking an aspirin every day is likely to prevent heart attacks and strokes, *or* it isn't.

- Vitamin E reduces the risk of heart disease, *or* it doesn't.

- Coronary stents prevent heart attacks, *or* they don't.

- Amyloid plaque causes Alzheimer's, *or* it doesn't and, in fact, it may be beneficial.[24]

- One of the most widely impactful reversals was on the efficacy of hormone replacement therapy (HRT). For decades HRT had been routinely prescribed for menopausal women before a 2002 Women's Health Initiative study found its risks outweighed its benefits so dramatically, that the study had to be stopped midstream to protect the subjects receiving HRT.[25]

Studies and Complementary and Alternative Medicine

Even if researchers are untouched by bias, concern for professional acceptance and reputation, or a desire for their study to meet significance-testing standards, and even if they are financially and technically capable of executing a well-designed study free of vulnerability and distorting influences, this kind of study is probably not an optimal way to assess the value of CAM practices.

Many CAM modalities address the complex reality and needs of individual patients, and tailor treatments accordingly. Because of this, even perfectly executed Western-style, double-blind studies are not suited to testing truly holistic medical modalities. If, for example, we test the efficacy of a designated dose of a particular medicine on every person in a study, this does not accurately represent or test how a truly holistic modality would either administer the medicine or treat the patient. If we want useful studies of these types of modalities, broader outcome-based studies would be more appropriate. For example, we could take X number of people who suffer from migraines and treat half of them with Ayurveda, TCM, or some other CAM modality. The rest would be given no treatment, or perhaps a placebo. This might offer more meaningful results.

But even outcome-based studies will not guarantee that a particular modality or remedy will work for the patient sitting in front of us. As individuals, we consume thousands of nutrients, in many forms, from various sources and countries. We exist in constantly shifting circumstances, climates, and relationships with each other and with the environment. The diverse influences we invite and to which we are exposed create a sort of network. When we change one factor, it affects the entire network. Even with the best-designed, best-executed, and most conclusive study, we cannot know the effect that any given therapy will have on any given patient.

However, while we may not learn from a study whether or not a particular remedy or therapy will be good for a particular patient, we may well learn something of the nature of the remedy or therapy, and that can be very helpful for increasing our theoretical knowledge.

If we see, for example, that ginger is shown to be effective in cases where cold is prevalent, we may understand that it is likely to have an inherent heating quality, and develop confidence in its use in cold conditions.

Reflections

When we take all this into consideration, "evidence-based medicine" seems an optimistic label for medical protocols dictated by study results. When misconduct affects research in every field of medicine, when positive findings are twice as likely to be published as negative ones, and when 50 percent of all study results are buried, suppressed, or go missing,[26] how can we, as doctors, trust the studies we read, or feel confident in the likely effects of the medicine we prescribe?

We saw earlier that Charaka advises us to discount testimony of those who are attached. This includes attachment to outcome. If research is tainted by significance chasing, bias, or financial incentive, or driven by the desire to have it published, this pretty much adds up to manipulating studies in order to support a particular outcome to which the designers are attached, and we cannot consider this a valid form of testimony, nor of knowledge.

With all the imperfections in modern research, there may still be value in it. If we question authority, consider who benefits from the results (financially or otherwise), and take those results under advisement, we may ultimately be better informed than if we either ignore the findings or treat them as gospel. We can generally place greater trust in results of studies wherein there is no huge financial beneficiary. We may also be able to place greater trust in results that reflect common sense. As James L. Mills, Chief of Pediatric Epidemiology at the National Institute of Child Health and Human Development, says, "A lot of findings that don't withstand the test of time didn't really make any sense in the first place."[27]

I like studies. I find that reading them and considering them help kindle my curiosity and interest in whatever herb, remedy, or therapy is being studied, and in the medical process itself.

Another, perhaps unintended, benefit of perusing studies may be that it builds confidence. If we become convinced of the beneficial effects of a remedy or therapy, *whether or not it is indeed efficacious,* our very confidence may have a beneficial effect on our patients and their outcome. A doctor's belief in a positive outcome for a patient can be an important factor in the success of treatment. More about that later.

In this book, I quote studies. Most of the studies I quote, and most of the ones I value in general, are those that seem motivated by scientific curiosity with no clear financial beneficiaries (aside from the consumers or patients). Those studies could be wrong, of course. Knowing the problems that plague both research and human nature, I could choose to ignore all studies, but I prefer to cultivate the approach taken by Dr. Kim A. Williams, President of the American College of Cardiology.

Dr. Williams adopted a vegan diet to reduce his cholesterol. It worked. Though he personally experienced a positive result, he acknowledged that many studies that demonstrate a positive correlation between diet and cholesterol levels (or diet and some other factor, for that matter) are observational. "There is a long list of things that, based on observational trials, we thought were beneficial, and then a randomized trial done for a long period of time showed that it wasn't," said Dr. Williams. "So I approach all of this with a sense of humility and an open mind."[28]

Our love affair with studies yields dubious value. Study results on herbs, therapies, or dietary factors do not equal knowledge. They add up to information that needs to be attended to with curiosity and skepticism. In the end, we still need to make our own best judgment, given the context, the patient, the disease, the stage and strength of the disease vs. the patient, and other influential factors.

The take-home message here may be: enjoy reading the study results, especially those that make sense and are not motivated by financial profit, but proceed with caution. Statistics, professors, textbooks, and other books may tell us something about a disease, a remedy, or a therapy, but they tell us nothing about the unique person sitting in front of us—the one who has the disease, takes the remedy, or uses the therapy.

2 Perception

Refining Our Ability to Perceive Knowledge

When you reach the end of what you should know,
you will be at the beginning of what you should sense.
KHALIL GIBRAN

Perception is that which is acquired with the
sense organs and mind directly.
CHARAKA[1]

Knowledge derived from the contact of self, sense
organs, mind, and sense objects, is explicit, and limited
to the present. It is known as perception.
CHARAKA[2]

Deciding a course of action becomes faultless if the disorder is
examined with the threefold sources of knowledge collectively,
because no knowledge is derived about the entire object by
a part of its source. Of these three sources of knowledge,
knowledge is obtained first from authority. Thereafter
examination proceeds with perception and inference...
CHARAKA[3]

Once we have learned theory from either a real or perceived authority—a source of information outside ourselves—it is time to turn to ourselves. Perception comes from us. Beyond clinical observation, questioning, and palpation taught in medical training, we can cultivate a more subtle ability to perceive. And this may be the most important thing we can do to cultivate the art of medicine. The more we refine our perceptive abilities, the better able we are to diagnose, and the more we nourish qualities central to the art of medicine.

Knowledge acquired by perception is pretty much the definition of empiricism—the theory that knowledge arises primarily from sensory experience—that is, what we perceive with our five senses. From a certain point of view, what we see, hear, taste, feel, and smell add up to what we know, and what we don't perceive adds up to what we don't know.

Empirical medical treatment is treatment based on practical experience or observation, rather than the scientific method, and we employ it regularly in all medical modalities. An example in Western medicine is when antibiotics are prescribed before a diagnosis is confirmed. The physician prescribes medicine based on empirical evidence—what she sees, hears, feels, and so on—rather than waiting for lab results to confirm a problem.

Few CAM practices rely on reading results of blood, saliva, and bodily fluid tests, or imaging tests routinely used in Western medicine, and instead rely heavily on personal observation. Relying so heavily on our senses necessitates their refinement. As it turns out, there is a happy side effect of doing so. When we refine our senses and perceptive abilities, we are not only better able to acquire knowledge, but we also refine our ability to communicate with patients—not an insignificant aspect of treatment.

The Subjectivity of Empiricism

Science and medicine, as well as common sense, recognize that our senses have limitations and can fool us. To circumvent these limitations, we may rely on statistical analyses of large groups of patients and the resulting numerical data to aid in our quest for knowledge. But even then we find it hard to escape the influence of our perceptions on how we design, execute, and implement studies in order to avoid biased results. As we have seen, double-blind studies may not be any less flawed, biased, or limited than our own perceptions.

While it may be hard to avoid limitations in any form of knowledge-gathering, perception is no less a valid form of knowledge than that gleaned from randomized tests or other sources of information. Neuroscientist V. S. Ramachandran, M.D., Ph.D., recounts a story and raises a question.[4] The story goes something like this: I bring you a talking pig. The pig asks after your welfare and what you think of the most recent Red Sox win (I am making up this part).

That's it. That's the story.

Not a gripping narrative, but the related question is: Do you need to see 100 or 100,000 more talking pigs to know that one exists? You do not. No more than you need to see the results from 100,000 other people in order to confirm overwhelming empirical evidence provided by the person in front of you.

One of the reasons we need huge studies in the first place is because often effects are so rare that it requires huge numbers of participants to discover statistically significant results. For example, if only three out of 100,000 people might experience a particular benefit or side effect from a given therapy, we would need to study many hundreds of thousands of people to detect that marginally statistically significant benefit or side effect. However, if the results are readily apparent to our perceptions, a small study based on empirical evidence—like a single talking pig—will be sufficient.

When empirical evidence is overwhelming, we do not need teachers or tests to confirm the results. For example, research on the benefits of mostly vegetable diets on heart disease is so conclusive that huge studies are not required. We can also see this evidenced in the origins of now-standard treatments, like the rabies vaccine or the use of extracorporeal membrane oxygenation (ECMO) machines that provide breathing and heart support for infants.

Before 1885, anyone who developed symptoms of rabies died from it. On July 6, 1885, a nine-year-old boy who had been bitten by a rabid dog, and who was at the highest risk for developing symptoms, was treated with a ten-day course of a rabies vaccine developed in Louis Pasteur's laboratory after extensive testing on animals. The boy survived and lived for many years. Thanks to his and one other case, the empirical results (everyone could see that they survived) were so clear that some three months later, it was decided that the vaccine should be made available for the public. By 1888, 1200 people had used the vaccine, with a mortality rate of 1 percent.[5] Death by rabies is a fearsome sentence and a gruesome end. Nobody would have been willing to be the one in the study who didn't get the vaccine.

In a more amusing example, Gordon Smith and Jill Pell wrote a satirical article in 2003 in which they pointed out that the use of parachutes was never subject to a randomized controlled trial. It was sufficient to observe that people without parachutes who survived falls from airplanes were rather thin on the ground.[6]

If we ignore one kind of evidence—say, empirical evidence—in favor of another—say, randomized, double-blind studies—we can pay high costs. Consider this example.

In the 1970s, ECMO was a revolutionary treatment for babies born with immature lungs. Its use substantially reduced infant mortality rates overnight. With such dramatic results, doctors didn't want to conduct a randomized control trial, especially because the babies in the control groups would almost certainly die. But they felt compelled to conduct such a trial, lest the scientific community ignore their results, claiming there was no large study to validate them. The researchers stopped the trial, however, after the fourth baby in the control group died, while nine out of nine of the babies receiving ECMO survived.[7]

A current example is the rapid rise of fecal transplants or fecal pills to treat Clostridium difficile infection (CDI). This rise is due to a 90 percent success rate.[8] Even though no massive studies have been conducted, results are so conclusive that we are adopting the protocol.

Thomas Hughes, L.Ac., a friend and colleague of mine, recently observed that we are each living a unique experiment. Since each of us is conceived, formed, born, grown, and nourished in different environments, relationships, foods, qualities, and proclivities, even the medicine most tailored to individuals, cannot perfectly conform to their unique constellation of influences and conditions. Though it is difficult—perhaps impossible—to perceive all these influences and conditions, if we hone our perceptive abilities, we have a better chance of perceiving more of them and matching the appropriate therapy with the patient in front of us.

Our perceptions about this unique, single patient may be more valuable than the results of studies on hundreds of other patients.

The five sensory abilities that feed our perceptions are seeing, hearing, smelling, tasting, and touching. Because touching, seeing, and hearing are most applicable to the skill sets of CAM practitioners, let us focus on these.

Refining Our Ability to Feel or Touch

Many of us spend our whole lives running from feeling with the mistaken belief that you cannot bear the pain. But you have already borne the pain. What you have not done is feel all you are beyond that pain.
KHALIL GIBRAN

Beyond physical palpation, we can cultivate the ability to feel the whole state of our patient—that is, their spirit, level of tension, disease, and wellbeing. One of the ways we can cultivate this ability is to refine our awareness of the sensations in our own bodies and beings.

In a curious University of Iowa study,[9] participants were each given four decks of cards, two blue and two red. They were instructed to turn over any card from any of the decks, and to do so one card at a time. Each card delivered either points or a penalty. The object of the game was twofold: to accumulate the most points and to determine which color cards—blue or red—would ultimately allow them to do so. What the participants didn't suspect until they had turned over about 50 cards (and couldn't confirm until they'd turned over about 80) was that, while the red cards sometimes rewarded the player with many points, they more often delivered bigger penalties. In the long run, the only way to win was by favoring the blue decks, which yielded fewer points, but smaller penalties.

The remarkable thing was that by the time the participants had turned over their tenth card, their *bodies* had already figured this out. Without any conscious awareness that red cards were the wrong choice, participants exhibited signs of stress (like increased sweat on their palms) when they pulled cards from the red decks—something they were already doing less of. This suggests that our bodies may be quicker to recognize trouble and discern truth than our conscious brains.

If we could cultivate our perceptive abilities and apply them to our own bodily sensations, perhaps our unconscious perceptions about the patient in front of us could more quickly become conscious.

It is my experience that they do. Once we feel ourselves, we are able to feel or sense the wellbeing of our patients more keenly. It is a little like this: when we know how to ride a bike, we know better how someone might feel as we watch them ride. And if we really are paying attention, we can feel where or when they may be feeling pain or pleasure. (To cultivate these abilities, we can practice visualizations like the one on page 55.)

We can cultivate this kind of subtle ability to feel. We can also cultivate less subtle abilities related to the sense of touch, like palpation and pulse-taking skills (if these are within our scope of practice). This improves our diagnostic abilities and, therefore, the chances of positive outcomes for our patients.

There are other more generalized and appropriate forms of touch, like hugging, hand shaking, or briefly placing a hand on the shoulder or arm of a patient, which can also serve to communicate empathy.

Studies have shown that a certain amount of touch—between one and three physical contacts like a pat on the back or handshake—during a patient visit significantly enhances a patient's trust in the doctor's empathy. My friend and colleague, Dr. Eduardo Cardona-Sanclemente, is aware of the value of appropriate, loving, physical touch. He says, "When patients come to me, the first thing they say is, 'Doctor you didn't give me my hug.' And I say, 'Yes. I am sorry.' Because that hug is a real acknowledgement that another human being is there in front of you who came to share his or her suffering."[10]

On the other hand, too much touch—more than three instances, according to studies—tends to backfire, communicating less empathy, perhaps because the touches feel forced, or even invasive.[11]

While it may seem contrived to formally study the magic number of touches that work to create rapport with a patient, it does require sensitivity to know whether touch will be perceived as appropriate or warranted. When I am aware of my own bodily sensations, I can sense when I've touched someone once too often. When this happens, it is often because I forgot to pay attention to my own internal compass and sensations, which would have alerted me that more touch was not a good idea. I recognize my mistake, usually silently, forgive myself, and move on. Trust can be regained.

I find that pulse taking, if that is part of the scope of practice, is a particularly valuable tool in the realm of touch. It is an intimate and safe experience, not to be hurried, and can create trust as well provide valuable clinical information.

Touch does not necessarily need to be physical. We can feel with other parts of ourselves than our fingertips and skin. We can feel our patients' wholeness, health, and condition with our wholeness, awareness, and directed attention. We feel not only their physical body, but also their energy and reality—we could call this their energetic body or reality. We join with them for this time, to feel what they are feeling in these bodies.

Dr. Cardona-Sanclemente puts it this way: "When I'm in front of a patient, I really try to participate with that human being, keeping that…connection between bodies while my intellect is trying to understand the physiological and pathological aspects. At the same time, I'm trying to sense how the different parts of the self are combined to manifest that particular imbalance or pathology."[12]

Touch, whether physical or empathic, yields a deeper, non-verbal form of communication with patients.

It feels to me that, when we feel or touch someone on a deep level, it is related to seeing and hearing deeply as well. Kirpal Singh ji Maharaj, a 20th-century saint in India, wrote that we receive 88 to 95 percent of our sensory impressions through what we see and hear. If true, this makes our ability to see and hear of particular significance to the practitioner.

Refining Our Ability to See

What we do see depends mainly on what we look for… In the same field, the farmer will notice the crop, the geologists the fossils, botanists the flowers, artists the colouring, sportsmen the cover for the game. Though we may all look at the same things, it does not all follow that we should see them.
JOHN LUBBOCK

Learn to see…accustom the eye to calmness, to patience, and to allow things to come up to it.
FRIEDRICH NIETZSCHE

After consulting many doctors and receiving many treatments to no avail, a man came to my guru for treatment. The man was suffering greatly with severe diarrhea, which he had endured for about a year. My guru put his hand on the man's head and told him that there was a blockage in his large intestine. He gave the man a strong laxative, which removed the blockage, and the man was fine after a couple days. Without the use of X-rays or even taking the man's pulse, my guru was able to "see" the man's problem.[13] This kind of ability, he said, is the product of experience and a result of engaging in spiritual practices.

My guru was not seeing with his two eyes. He was using his internal vision. This is a level of seeing that goes beyond what formal medical training usually teaches us to observe. Whether or not we can develop that level of refinement, we can certainly find ways to improve our abilities. It may be helpful to understand that our starting point—how and what we perceive now—is likely a product of our history and environment. Once we know this, we can begin to cultivate a more open mind and refined abilities.

Studies strongly suggest that environment and functional demand can determine behavioral and physiological perception. In a study on cats, for example, researchers found that cats raised in an environment rich with vertical lines (but devoid of horizontal ones) grew up "blind" to horizontal lines, and vice versa.[14] While this study was on the physical ability to see, the same may be true for our non-physical ability. We may be especially vulnerable to environmental influences on our perceptive abilities in utero and during the early years of life but, throughout our lives, what we see, the importance we attach to it, and the meaning we derive from it may be influenced by our environment and culture.

There is a story (variously and erroneously attributed to Darwin, Magellan, or Columbus) that occurred during Captain Cook's 1770 landing in Australia. The story is often misreported, too, claiming that although the aboriginal people could see the canoes the explorers used to come ashore, they were unable to see the large ship upon which they arrived. The accepted conclusion is that the big boat was so beyond the experience of the indigenous people, that they were literally unable to see it.

This is a fascinating idea because, as in the case with the cats, it suggests that we humans also cannot see what we are not conditioned to see. Fascinating idea, and one that holds up even if we get the Captain Cook story right.

Upon close examination of the accounts of Joseph Banks, the botanist who travelled with Captain Cook, and of the captain himself, it appears more likely that the aborigines were simply not concerned with the foreigners until they made attempts to come ashore, at which point they tried to drive the explorers away. There was actually plenty of evidence that they did, in fact, see the big ship but didn't react until they felt threatened.

Ironically, the aboriginal response was surprising to Captain Cook and his men because it was outside *their* experience. When they first approached Alaska, for example, the native people there canoed out to meet and welcome them in friendship. When the explorers arrived in New Zealand, the Maoris, too, reacted quickly, if less warmly, canoeing toward their big ship—brandishing spears and threatening attack. The surprising thing for Cook and his men was that the Australian aborigines did not take much notice of or make a fuss about their ship. This does not mean that they did not see it. They simply neither welcomed the explorers nor felt threatened by them until the new arrivals encroached too closely on their territory.[15]

The actual story conveys a noteworthy idea: what each of us perceives may not hold equal significance or fascination for another, and may, in part, be a product of our environment, culture, and experience.

The aboriginals were unconcerned—or only peripherally concerned—with the large ship, until the intruders began to violate their cultural (and geographical) boundaries. The Maoris' territory may have extended into deeper waters, and thus their communal response was to strike out sooner. The Alaskans had yet a different reaction. Each of the native people's cultures and environments influenced what they perceived to be important or threatening.

This is worthwhile to keep in mind for several reasons. One is that we need to remember that what *we* think is important to focus and act on is, at least in part, a conclusion based on the conditioning of our own environment and culture: it may not be The Truth.

Another point is that patients from various cultures may have the same apparent circumstances or disorders, but have wildly different prognoses according to their unique cultural influences. For example, an elopement or a falling out between a son or daughter and their parents may carry different weight and ramifications for someone born and raised in a traditionally Eastern culture vs. a Western one. These events may cause minor discord in the latter, yet have massive consequences in the former. The stress experienced by patients from these differing backgrounds will likely be radically different, affecting treatment strategy and possibly prognosis.

Even within a single culture, there are wide ranges of stressors that can affect diagnosis and outcomes—factors like lifestyle stressors, financial pressure, number of hours worked in a week, and how much support we receive. If we don't see the patient's physical, familial, and cultural context, we may miss important influences. Norman Sartorius of the World Health Organization (WHO) goes so far as to say, "Social factors play a major and important role in the outcome of disease. Very few solutions are medical in medicine."[16] It is because of this that, after being in practice for a number of years, I added a question to my initial intake process: *What are your main stressors, and your main sources of support?* This would give me an idea if the stressors were outweighing the support system, and would be a factor in the prognosis. It helped me see the bigger picture—the context in which the patient was living her life and suffering her ailments.

While our physical vision, as we saw with the cats, may be hardwired a certain way thanks to our early environment, and while the things we perceive to be important are influenced by our culture and environment, it is also true that both our physical ability to see, and our subtle ability to perceive reality, are malleable. We can develop, change, and refine them. Even if we are blind.

John Hull, the blind author of *Touching the Rock: An Experience of Blindness*, developed the ability to be, "a whole-body seer."[17] Once the 17th-century poet John Milton became blind, he meditated on the process of inward sight replacing outward sight.[18] When Zoltan Torey became blind at 21, he resolved to develop his inner visual ability. He became so adept at this that he could imagine himself inside the inner workings of machines and systems.[19] Clinical psychologist and psychotherapist, Dr. Dennis Shulman, applies this ability to his patients. He finds he is better aware of their emotional conditions since becoming blind. He can sense their subtle levels of tension or anxiety, and finds the sounds of their voices and even their smells reveal their depths.[20] One of the things happening here is, when the visual cortex is not being constantly activated by external stimuli, it becomes more sensitive to internal and other stimuli—stimuli like signals from our sensory input, and even our thoughts and emotions.[21] We do not need to go blind to refine our internal sight, but we do need to pay close attention.

Consider the Moken (also called the Sea Gypsies) of Southeast Asia. To the Moken, the ocean is their universe. For most of the year, they live traditionally on hand-built wooden boats, migrating between islands as their needs and patterns of nature dictate. Before the great Sumatra-Andaman earthquake of 2004 created the infamous tsunami, the Moken saw dolphins begin to swim for deeper water. They noticed elephants beginning to stampede to higher ground, and they heard the cicadas fall silent. When they saw and heard these things, they knew danger was imminent, and they either sailed to the deep sea or retreated to high ground. They all survived the tsunami.

When the Moken later heard that squid fishers in the sea had perished because they had no foreknowledge of impending trouble, one Sea Gypsy observed, "They were looking at squid. They were not looking at anything. They saw nothing, they looked at nothing. They don't know how to look."[22] The squid fishers might have seen the same things that the Moken saw but, even if they did, they were unable to perceive the importance of them, to realize they meant trouble was coming.

Even the Moken's visual organs have adapted to their depth of vision. Their visual acuity is so refined that that they can control the shape of their ocular lenses and the size of their pupils when necessary.[23]

We can find a more cosmopolitan but equally striking example of this sort of cultivation of the senses in the famous story of the authentication of the Getty kouros (kouroi are archaic Greek statues of young, healthy, usually naked, men)—a statue acquired by the J. Paul Getty Museum in Malibu, California. Though at the time of purchase in 1985 the kouros had been "proven" to be genuine, based largely on a scientific surface chemistry test,[24] experts who had spent their professional lives observing such sculptures declared almost instantly that the statue was not, in fact, authentic. To this day, even after subsequent investigation, neither art historians nor scientists have been able to conclusively establish its authenticity.[25]

How did the experts recognize the ambiguity so quickly? Maybe it works something like this: when we focus on a subject, like art or medicine, for a long time, each bit of related data that we memorize, see, hear, feel, or otherwise ingest into the macro computer that is our brain and consciousness is stored. Then, when we have a statue or patient in front of us, and "input" their appearance and symptoms into our macro computer, it is able to "output" useful information, like knowledge of veracity or a diagnosis that relates to the pathology.

In Daoism there is a term called *nei kuan*, or "inner vision." If we employ inner vision, we can "see" what is happening in our patients. Not literally, but with our mind's eye, as in the story of my guru and the man with the blockage in his intestine. This is what is happening, maybe to a slightly lesser extent, when very experienced physicians know what is wrong with their patients within minutes of being with them. We can cultivate *nei kuan* by learning to visualize the activities, flow, directionality, and function of the various organs, tissues, and energies of the body.

This is one of the benefits of naming organs and patterns of pathology. Labels like "Liver qi stagnation," or "*vata* in the *majjavahasrotas*" are not reality. They are terms employed to describe reality, so that we can better picture it in our mind's eye. They allow us to organize a constellation of physical, mental, and emotional symptoms, appearances, observations, smells, sounds, textures, and even tastes into a pattern that explains their connection and serves to point us in the direction of the root cause.

Without learning to see patterns like this, we would run the risk of analysis paralysis—a syndrome associated with the phenomenon of over-analysis, which paralyzes our ability to arrive at an elegant diagnosis. When we equally weight all symptoms and observations, our diagnosis can be confused and complicated, making it harder to choose an effective treatment plan. We may collect mounds of seemingly disparate information about a patient, but the patterns and paradigms of thought we have previously learned somehow sort all that information into a pattern, even if we are not conscious of the sorting process. I have found that the only sure way to know what to focus on and what symptoms to weight more heavily than others, is to practice—to see many patients for many years. That takes time, of course. But if we are focusing on our patients and doing the best we can, we are already in the process of refining our ability to see what is important.

Some aspects of seeing do not have to wait for practice. One straightforward aspect of the visual sense organ at work is simple eye contact. Eye contact has proven to inspire such powerful feelings of connection that companies use this in their advertising to influence us—and our children. For example, the characters on cereal boxes are created to look directly at us—or down a little to simulate eye contact with children looking up at them in the supermarket aisle.[26]

Studies have shown that eye contact, like touch, significantly enhances a patient's trust in a doctor's empathy and communication skills.[27] Indeed, it is so powerful that even when people are blind, their brains respond to eye contact.[28]

Eye contact activates parts of the brain that allow us to more accurately perceive another person's feelings and intentions,[29] but, as with the amount of appropriate touch, there is a comfort zone. Some is very good, but too much tends to break the trust or feel forced.[30] Consider the line between looking intently and staring. The former can inspire a feeling of connection, while the latter can feel creepy, forced, disingenuous, or even intimidating.

Sometimes looking directly into someone's eyes invades their privacy. I recently read about a man who spent 27 years alone, living in a tent in the woods of Maine, without having even one conversation with another human being in the entire time. When he came out, he found it difficult to maintain eye contact. He explained, "I'm not used to seeing people's faces. There's too much information there. Aren't you aware of it? Too much, too fast."[31] Clearly, to look directly into this man's eyes would violate his privacy.

While perhaps none of our patients have lived the life of a hermit, it is still worthwhile to consider whether eye contact is appropriate or necessary for someone to feel seen in an accurate and whole way.

In fact, it is worth asking whether direct eye contact is always necessary in order to see someone effectively. My guru actually used to counsel his disciples *not* to look directly into the eyes of other people, but rather, to look between and slightly above, their eyes. Even without gazing into someone's eyes, it is possible to feel a real contact that involves seeing and connecting with the whole being. When we look into someone's eyes, we are communicating that we are taking time to fully see them and that we care enough to do so. But this may be accomplished without actually looking into someone's eyes. Simply being with them and connecting with them with our whole being may accomplish a similar effect. We see with more than our eyeballs. We see with our brains and perceive with our whole beings.

Finally, we can train our sights to focus on and see the Good and the Divine in each of our patients. In Eastern medicine we learn that where our attention goes, *prana*—life force—follows. When we pay attention to the Good, we feed it. As Alex Haley says, "Find the good and praise it!" *Simply looking for or seeing the spark of the Divine in another feeds it*, no matter how dim (or strong) the spark may be. This, in itself, may have therapeutic benefit.

While there are doubtless limitations to perception, we can learn to cultivate it so that we can see and communicate with our patients more deeply and creatively, a combination that will yield a greater understanding of the patient, his condition, empathy, and the powerful healing possibilities.

Refining Our Ability to Hear and Speak

Listen to the wind, it talks. Listen to the silence,
it speaks. Listen to your heart, it knows.
NATIVE AMERICAN PROVERB

As with feeling, touching and seeing, there are physical, mechanical aspects of hearing and speaking, as well as more subtle aspects of hearing and communicating. Both aspects can, and probably often do, co-exist.

Many of us listen to a patient's history selectively. We listen for certain signs or symptoms that may confirm a suspected diagnosis. This is good, but if that is all we listen for, we can miss other important parts of their story. And miss hearing what is unspoken.

When we speak, sound comes from us. When we hear, it comes to us. What we say and hear, then, are two sides of the same experience, like feeling and touching. In fact, in the Sanskrit language, I have seen the words *shabdha*, meaning sound, and *vani*, meaning speech, used somewhat interchangeably when it comes to categories of communication through speech and hearing. Let us look a little closer.

Indian philosophical systems describe two categories of sound: *dhun atmak shabda* and *varn atmak shabda*.[32] *Dhun atmak shabda* can be described as that internal sound that enlivens all beings and from which we all arise. It is synonymous with "the Word" of Judeo-Christian tradition or the concepts of divine sound present in many, if not all, other religions. It is the "unstruck sound," the sound of one hand clapping—a sound not created by duality—that is, by one thing striking another.

It is the less subtle, second type of sound, *varn atmak shabda,* through which the *atma* or soul expresses itself and functions in this physical world of five elements. It is this type of sound that is relevant to our conversation here.

Varn atmak shabda relates to both verbal and non-verbal language. We employ it when we relay and receive information, ideas, and emotions, and communicate in general with other human beings or with any sentient beings or species. We also use it in prayer. As with touch and sight, sound can be external or internal; it can be audible or inaudible. We hear with more than our ears and communicate with more than our tongues.

Varn atmak shabda can be broken into four categories of *shabda* (sound or speech), or *vani* (speech).[33] I find these apply to both hearing and speaking, as one receives and the other transmits sound. The four categories are:

- *Vaikari vani* or *shabdha*, performed by tongue, out loud.

- *Madhyma vani* or *shabdha,* performed mentally, at the seat of the throat.

- *Pashyanti vani* or *shabdha*, performed silently, from the seat of the heart.

- *Para vani* or *shabdha*, also a silent process, performed from the seat of the navel.

When we communicate with our patients, or in any relationship, we can consider which *vani* or type of speech we are employing. For example, how often do we say something with our tongue but without our thoughts, hearts, or attention committed to the communication? With each successive and deeper level of communication, we find increasing integrity in communication—integrity being defined as an undivided state of wholeness where all levels of communication are aligned. There may be other ways of understanding the flavor and nature of each of these types of communication, but here are my personal reflections on them.

Vaikari Vani

Vaikari vani is the spoken word or vocalizations. Without it, we would have no vocal way to convey or record emotions, thoughts, or prescriptions. It is possible to convey either meaningful ideas through *vaikari vani,* or very little of substance. We can make meaningless sounds with our mouths or tongues—clicking noises, whistling, scatting—or another noise that may seem or be meaningless, or meaningful. They may signify truth, untruth, or something in between. For example, we walk down the street, meet someone we know, and say, "Hey, how are ya?" and keep walking, without really caring to know, in fact, how they actually are. We have communicated something in words but without aligning it with genuine thought, emotion, or attention. This type of communication is famously employed in cocktail parties, where it is possible to spend an entire evening engaged in brief conversations, and come away not having really learned or communicated anything meaningful with anyone, including ourselves.

When we communicate with words alone, we may not be as helpful to our patients as when we take the time to align our words with deeper levels of meaning.

Madhyama Vani

Madhyama vani arises from the throat and is related to thoughts. We may choose to align our thoughts with our tongues or not. If we take that same example of walking down the street and meeting someone when we are in a hurry, if we say, "Hey, how are ya?" while our thoughts are *Oh no, it is someone I know, and I have to get to the bookstore before it closes*, our thoughts and words are not in alignment. If we chose to align them, we might add, "I am in a bit of a hurry to get to the bookstore before it closes."

Needless to say, it is not necessary or even desirable to speak every thought we have. That may be hurtful. But generally, the tenets of ethical living enjoin us to tell the truth. How to reconcile these two sometimes seemingly incompatible states? Kirpal Singh, a 20th-century saint in India, used to say that, before we speak, it is useful to ask ourselves if what we are about to say is true, kind, and necessary. If it is not *all three*, he advised, it may be better left unsaid. In order to have our thoughts and words in alignment and also to be kind, we may need to discipline our thoughts.

My teacher used to tell this story. Emperor Akbar had heard that one's thoughts about others have a strong effect on them, and he wanted to see an example of this. One of his advisors suggested they do an experiment. They stood in the road and saw a man at a great distance, walking towards them. The advisor asked the Emperor what he was thinking when he saw the man, who turned out to be a farmer. Emperor Akbar did not know the farmer, but confessed he had had the thought *I should have him killed.* He had no reason to entertain this thought, but it arose nonetheless. When the farmer approached, Emperor Akbar, obeying his advisor, asked the farmer to tell him what he thought when he saw it was the Emperor who was standing in the road. To encourage honesty, he assured the farmer no ill would come to him as a result of telling the truth. The farmer admitted that when he saw the Emperor, he wanted to pound the Emperor's bare head with his fists. This is how Emperor Akbar became convinced that our thoughts influence the very thing upon which they are focused.

Our private thoughts while we are with our patients may have a beneficial or negative effect on them, depending on what these thoughts are. If we truly aim to "do no harm," we must also aim to have disciplined thoughts.

The question may arise, what about the effect of patients' thoughts on us? Some practitioners claim to feel drained at the end of a day of treating patients, exhausted beyond the fatigue commensurate with the hours worked. We consider this later, in Chapter 34. Whether this is a result of our patients' thoughts or not, for now it is enough to consider our own thoughts.

Pashyanti Vani

The truth that we can heal, we must learn again. Medicine is in our hearts and also in the heart of that which we call the Universe.
NIKOLA TESLA

Kirpal Singh taught that man speaks from the abundance of his heart. If we are not connected to our hearts, we may simply speak our minds. Expressing ourselves from our hearts—practicing *pashyanti vani*—requires that we be aware of feelings that color the present moment.

One woman who publicly discusses the value of communication from the heart and seems to have cultivated this skill to an impressive degree is Anna Breytenbach. Breytenbach calls herself an "interspecies communicator," and offers seminars and workshops to help others do the same. While talking with animals may sound farcical at first, when we watch Breytenbach in active communication with an animal, it is hard to argue with her authenticity. One example of her work was portrayed in a moving 13-minute video entitled, "The incredible story of how leopard Diabolo became Spirit,"[34] in which Breytenbach demonstrates an ability to communicate with an angry and reclusive black leopard, dramatically altering his mental health and behavior. This YouTube video seems to have spoken to the heart of many two-legged creatures as well: It went viral, garnering some 1.5 million views within five months of being posted.

In one of her newsletters,[35] Anna describes a technique for people to begin to communicate with animals in the way she does, whether the animal is present or far away. It is a process whereby you sit quietly, set an intention to have clear intuition, open your heart, visualize a connection between your heart and the animal's heart, call their name, and send them a greeting. Then you communicate what you want to know, ask, or tell them.

Breytenbach advises that we not be attached to any particular outcome with the animal, nor be in a hurry. Instead, we should remain patiently open to receiving communication the animal wishes to send. She says that she sends and receives communication through words that arise in her awareness, in visual images she sees internally, or in emotional or physical feelings. She stresses having patience and allowing plenty of time to become aware of any subtle communication you may be receiving. While Breytenbach teaches and practices subtle communication with animals, her technique can be applied to all humans, creatures, and plants with which we share our lives and our environment.

One of the potential pitfalls occurs when our hearts are overcrowded with emotion. While we don't want to be cold hearted with our patients, we may err in the other direction and indulge our emotions. Since emotions are forever in flux, they do not provide a stable foundation from which to communicate.

If our hearts are filled with emotion, we may pollute *pashyanti vani* and, rather than communicating with a clear heart, we may instead encourage waves of turbulent emotion in our relationships with our patients and others. Since we feed what we focus on, it is more stabilizing to focus on clarity in the heart, rather than emotions that may be roiling there. Then, when we speak and listen from a clear heart, we speak and listen with empathy instead of emotion.

Para Vani

Para vani is a form of communication that I find particularly beneficial. It is employed with our attention situated in the area of the navel or lower abdomen. This type of communication requires two things: first, the willingness to take the time to be present in the situation and moment; and second, the ability to breathe into the lower abdomen. This is something you may have heard about, perhaps in a yoga class, but have not yet practiced. People may even practice yoga for years and still not be confident that they know how to engage this type of breathing. (If you need help learning to breathe into the lower abdomen, try the simple exercise below.) If we can't breathe into the lower abdomen, it is impossible to communicate from it.

Cultivating Internal Awareness and Dissolving Obstructions

Sit in a comfortable position from which you will not need to move for about ten minutes. Allow your breath to become long and slow. Add a gentle pause at the top of the inhale and the bottom of the exhale.

Bring your awareness to your lower abdomen, from your pubic bone to your belly button. Allow each inhale to completely and smoothly fill this area, so that it expands with your breath, starting from the core of your being and moving out into its periphery. Take a gentle pause and then exhale, allowing your abdomen and breath to relax back to your core.

If it helps, you can place your hands gently over your abdomen or at its sides so you can feel your breath push out your belly when you inhale and relax when you exhale.

Once you have established this pattern, close your eyes, awaken your inner vision, and "look" around your lower abdomen for any tight, dark, or sticky spots. Once you identify a spot, direct your attention to it and imagine you are breathing into its center.

If you have trouble doing this, put your hand over the spot and imagine there is a straw going through your hand and penetrating the spot. Then breathe through the straw. As your breath enters the spot, see and feel the tightness, darkness, or stickiness dissolve.

Once you have dissolved one spot, switch your attention to another and repeat.

After a few minutes, shift your attention to the area between your belly button and just below your breasts, and repeat the process—allowing each inhale to completely and smoothly fill this area so it expands with your breath, starting from the core of your being and moving out into its periphery. Take a gentle pause and then exhale, allowing your abdomen and breath to relax back to your core. Then look for and dissolve any tight, dark, or sticky spots in this area.

Repeat this whole process once more in the area that spans from below your breasts up to your neck.

Finally, return your breath to the lower abdomen and finish up with a few full breaths into that area.[36]

Practicing *para vani* allows us to communicate with our whole being and be aware of the patient's whole being. While not discounting the words a patient is using, the thoughts they are expressing, or the emotions they are experiencing, these simply become threads in the greater fabric of the practitioner's total experience of who the patient is. This ability is not unique to human communication. When we watch animals size each other up, for example, it appears that they are communicating with each other without thought, words, or even emotions, but with their whole bodies.

In Ayurveda, we talk about each living being having a life force body (*pranamayakosha*), a physical body (*annamayakosha*), and a mental body (*manomayakosha*).[37] The life force body pervades the entire physical body and is intimately connected to the mental body. It feels to me that this is what I am communicating from and with when I employ *para vani*. This may sound abstract or esoteric, but to me it feels like a tangible and practical skill to cultivate.

When we use *para vani* to communicate with our patients, we cultivate a broader perspective, and a greater depth of understanding becomes possible. When we communicate this way, it may also serve as an example and invitation to our patients to do the same. We may find our patients begin their interactions with us with *vaikari vani*, then slowly settle into deeper levels of communication as they feel we are not in a hurry and that we want to hear them in the most complete way we can. We may even hear this shift reflected in the timbre of their voice, if it starts somewhat tight or high and gets more resonant or lower and more relaxed as time passes.

Achieving this type of communication, I find, cannot be rushed. If we are rushed, we are not fully present, and *para vani* is not possible unless we are fully present. Taking time with patients and being fully present with them conveys and reflects care. Not that we need a study to prove that this is important to our patients, but we do have them, and they demonstrate that this is so—and that this type of communication tends to improve patient compliance and therapeutic outcomes.[38]

I had a dear friend in India who, in my experience, excelled at *para vani*. We would sit together, wordlessly and without distraction or looking at each other for about five minutes. Then I might say something, and a minute or so would pass before he would say something. Sometimes a half hour or so would pass like this before we would move on to other activities or obligations. Though he has since passed away, the intimacy and depth of communication that flowed in those short meetings were, and remain, precious to me, and serve as a reminder of the depth and flavor of *para vani*.

Reflections

There is no intuitive determination in him who is uncontrolled,
And there is likewise no concentration in him who is uncontrolled,
And in him who does not concentrate, there is no peace.
Whence can come happiness to him who is not peaceful?
BHAGAVAD GITA: II: 66[39]

If the doors of perception were cleansed,
everything would appear to man as it is: Infinite.
WILLIAM BLAKE

We use our sense organs to perceive. If we have not controlled our senses, the *Gita* says, there is little chance for "intuitive determination." While I don't know what is meant by "intuitive determination," I feel that it indicates a kind of confidence in our intuition, which is fed by our senses. If our senses are clear, so too the intuition. If clouded, so too the intuition.

My guru told me that a doctor should be healthy herself and should be regular with her spiritual practices. One of the side effects of a regular daily spiritual practice is the purification of the senses. For example, focusing on a point or a candle serves to purify the visual sense, whether the eyes are open or closed. Focusing on a mantra or prayer purifies our tongue and ears, whether we sing, hear it with our ears, or hear it in our heads. Clearing the mind and heart of malice, judgment, attachment, and other strong emotions purifies the senses, which is necessary in order to feel, see, hear, and speak clearly.

Various Indian traditions have long placed great emphasis on refining, disciplining, and purifying the sense organs. I learned from my teachers that we can control or discipline each sense organ in numerous ways.

- We help purify the eyes by striving to see the good in others and by avoiding looking at anyone or anything with lust, anger, greed, attachment, or a desire to dominate or influence them or it. We can also engage in certain spiritual practices that refine our ability to see or focus on the divine or on an image that represents the divine.

- We help purify the ears by refusing to hear gossip or ugly speech. We can also use spiritual practices like listening to divine sound or to music that represents the divine, like hymns, prayers, kirtan, bhajan, or chants.

- We help purify the tongue by refusing to gossip or speak unkindly or dishonestly, or indulge in tasty food or drink to the detriment of our body. We can also speak sweetly and with love; eat and drink that which we know is healthful for us; and sing, chant, or recite prayers, mantras, or other uplifting sounds or words.

- We help purify the sense of touch by touching people with love and care rather than lust or violence. We can also focus on images of the Divine or nature that we can empathize with and become, to some degree.

- We help purify our sense of smell by *not* consuming something that smells delicious if we know it will not be good for us. (Sometimes smelling natural or fresh scents can also help in this regard.)

- With all of our senses, we can keep them physically healthy and clear as well—something that various medical traditions address in their unique ways.

The idea is, when our orifices and senses are purified and clear, we (as doctors and as individuals) will have a more beneficial effect on humanity, and humanity will have a more beneficial effect on us. When we discipline our desires—desires that arise in response to sensory stimuli—our life force changes momentum and direction. Rather than dissipating into a world of seductive and repulsive sights, sounds, tastes, sensations, and smells, our life force turns inward and concentrates. As it becomes contained within us, we feel strengthened, more content, more centered, and less fatigued. This can also have an effect on our patients.

Experience has shown that we humans have a tremendous ability to cultivate our perceptive abilities. Just as the Moken developed keen perceptive abilities, so can we, over time, and with practice.

As we seek knowledge through our perceptions, we can strive to go beyond our habitual and medically trained use of our senses. We can learn to feel, touch, see, and hear and communicate subtly and internally as well as with our external organs. As we are unlikely to clearly perceive what is going on in someone else if we can't clearly perceive what is going on in ourselves, we can start with ourselves. We can perceive our own inner sensations and reality. Then we can feel more than what we palpate, perhaps touch our patients' hearts, can see more than what is displayed, hear what is unspoken, and communicate using more than speech. Doing so gives us a deeper understanding of our patients, more empathy, and a greater ability to communicate.

As one blind person may work to cultivate their inner vision and another refine their sense of hearing to fill in their perception and experience of reality, the experience of activating and refining internal sensory experience for anyone may vary according to our nature. It may also be hard to separate out the various inner sensory experiences. I have found the experience of deeply and subtly touching to be similar to the experience of deeply and subtly feeling, seeing, hearing, or speaking. All these sensory experiences connect, relate, and comingle inside the brain, heart, and body. They become an entwined internal experience of cognition that, for me at least, is hard to describe. As with the four successively deeper types of speech, we can sense successively deeper with each sense. I return again to John Hull's description, "whole-body seer," but it is more accurate—for me—to say, "whole-body cognizer."

Sensory intermingling is true for physical sensory pathways as well. While true to some degree for everybody, it is why deaf people may experience lip reading as hearing, synesthetes see sounds or hear colors, and blind people may "see" the world through sensations.[40] Seeing, hearing, touching, smelling, and tasting are not separate, distinct neural pathways once they depart their orifices and organs and enter interior realms. They, too, intertwine to become a rich inner experience of cognition.

It may, in fact, be quite rare or impossible to have an experience purely of one single sense. Therefore, if we refine our ability to hear, for example, we may find ourselves better able to see and feel as well, whether we are talking about perceiving through our physical senses or more subtly, through our internal sensory apparatus. Whichever sense or senses we refine, cognition and communication improves.

And better communication is an excellent goal, not least because it is not always a doctor's strong suit. In one study, 75 percent of orthopedic surgeons—but only 21 percent of their patients—thought the doctor's communication was satisfactory.[41] One report suggests that 85 percent of patients either changed or considered changing physicians due to what the patients perceived as poor communication skills.[42] If this is an accurate indication, we have more than a little room for improvement.

Communication is not limited to what we say aloud. Non-verbal messaging has a powerful effect on the overall experience of communication, and on a patient's perception and experience (if not the doctor's experience) of empathy.

When we refine our senses and pay attention to a patient, empathy is invited into the relationship. There are studies that explore why this is, and the mechanisms for how this happens. For example, when we watch someone perform an action, like touching their nose, the same parts of our brains light up as when we touch our own nose (albeit to a lesser degree). Scientists theorize that this is one of the mechanisms that enables us to feel empathy. We will look at this in more depth in Part IV later. The fact that we experience the same thing that we see someone else experiencing, even if to a lesser degree, allows us to feel our patients' experience. In other words, empathy is a subtle form of perception, and therefore a side effect of refining our abilities to perceive.

The importance of the role empathy plays in treatment outcomes has been widely studied and shown to play a significant role. For example, Type 2 diabetes patients who perceived their doctors as empathic experienced far fewer complications—like hyperglycemia, excessively low insulin production, and even diabetic coma—than those treated by doctors perceived as minimally empathetic.[43]

There are actually efforts underway to find the sweet spot for the amount of non-verbal communication between doctor and patient. The goal is not purely humanitarian. Scientists hope to engineer systems and technologies that determine and encourage just the right amount of communication, thereby potentially increasing patient compliance (which is good for the patient), and reducing the likelihood that patients will seek out new doctors (which is bad for cost-control in the healthcare system).

It may be unnecessary to get academic about this and use systems that dictate how many seconds to engage in eye contact with a patient, or how many times to pat them on the back. If we are paying attention to our own internal compass and sensations, as discussed in the section on refining our ability to feel, we might actually be able to work this out for ourselves. On the other hand, if we have a hard time reading social cues, such seemingly academic information and systems might be useful.

The more effective the communication between doctor and patient, the more patient–doctor trust is fostered, and the more likely the two can agree on a treatment program. All of this adds up to a greater likelihood of a positive outcome.

Seeing with more than our eyes, hearing with more than our ears, feeling with more than our fingertips... It's all part of tapping into something deeper. It invites intimacy into the doctor–patient relationship and empathy into the healing process.

3 Inference

The Role of Prediction in Knowledge

Inference is based on prior perception. It is of three types and is related to the three times. One can infer covered fire from the smoke, sexual intercourse from observing the fetus, and the future fruit from a seed.
CHARAKA[1]

Once we have theoretical knowledge from valid authorities and have applied our own refined perceptions to a patient's case, it is time to employ inference, the last valid source of knowledge, according to Charaka.

Charaka writes that there are three types of inference, each of which can be represented best by a metaphor. The first is that we infer fire—even if we cannot see it—from the presence of smoke. The second is that we infer sexual relations from the presence of a fetus, and the third is that we infer an apple from an apple seed. We can see that the first relates to the present, the second to the past, and the third to the future. Inference relates to something in the past, present, or future that we have not witnessed first hand. It relates to the role of prediction in medicine. It is this trio of past, present, and future to which I believe Charaka is referring when he refers to "the three times" in the opening quote to this chapter. Inference is what ties them all together.

One of the great strengths of good medicine is its ability to stop a problem before it starts. This is truly preventive medicine as opposed to early detection. In order to stop a problem before it starts, though, we need to have a sense of the trajectory of the life of our patient. Using inference, we can take the patient's past and present into consideration in order to track the likely trajectory of their health and wellbeing to predict the future, and then change it, if necessary and possible.

In the modern world, I think it is easy to confuse early detection with prevention. They are decidedly not the same thing. If we detect breast cancer early, for example, there is still breast cancer. We have not prevented it.

One of the real strengths of Eastern medicine is true disease prevention. And to truly prevent disease, we need a kind of predictive ability.

We consider a patient's present condition, how virulent it is, take its inception and history into consideration, and we predict where they will be in X amount of time if their circumstances remain the same. Then, if the trajectory doesn't look good, we try to interrupt and redirect it.

We are attempting to look into the future. We are combining the patient's story with our own, guessing at an outcome, and trying to redirect the story, if needed. That's the job when it comes to preventive medicine. Anyone with a skeptical eye can see it's not an exact science. It is *a guess*. An inference. But the better we can be at inference—at prediction—the more potential we have to interrupt a negative trajectory or support a positive one. The better we are at prediction, the better the outcome, potentially.

Prediction is different than personal projection. We want to cultivate the former and avoid the latter. We don't want to see something so badly that we see it even where it does not exist. We want to purify our senses, as discussed, so that we may perceive things as they are, as much as possible, without attachment to how we want them to be or how we think they should be. But this does not mean we should avoid prediction.

The Present: Inferring Fire from Smoke

This metaphor refers to the present. If we see no fire, but we see smoke, we can infer that there must be a fire somewhere present now. We infer that certain diseases or conditions are present by looking at the patient's current signs and symptoms.

For example, in TCM, if we see a rash and irritability, we infer that the patient's Liver health, Lungs, or Blood might be compromised. If there are loose stools and fatigue, we infer that the patient's digestive system is taxed, even if a patient claims he has no problem with his digestion. We have to infer that there is fire, even when the patient is not aware of it and is only concerned about the smoke.

We want to be careful not to mistake the smoke for the fire, however. It may be tempting to think that the smoke itself is the problem (and certainly smoke can cause its own problems), but there is usually a root cause for a patient's symptoms. We do not find smoke without fire. Setting up a fan to blow the smoke away may alleviate the symptom of choking, but the fire will continue to burn.

Sometimes the root cause of the symptom is far from obvious. Let us take the example of the role of amyloid plaque in Alzheimer's. Amyloid is a common chemical structure produced by every cell in our body. It is also a major component of the plaque found to accumulate in the brains of patients with Alzheimer's and multiple sclerosis. For decades, the hypothesis in Western medicine was that amyloid was proinflammatory; it was a neurotoxin on which we could blame dementia.

However, when amyloid was studied further, the opposite was found to be true.[2] When researchers worked to eliminate amyloid plaque in patients with dementia, results were neutral at best. Sometimes the patients even got worse.[3] This led researchers to consider whether the amyloid plaque was actually serving a useful purpose. So they injected amyloid into mice that were paralyzed by multiple sclerosis. The mice regained their ability to walk. When the plaque was removed, the mice once again became paralyzed. This reinforced the hypothesis that the amyloid plaque was actually helping.

Let's step back a moment. We know that the body, with its innate intelligence, will often find ways to protect its vital organs, like the brain. So we could ask why, if amyloid plaque is harmful, it is being deposited in the brain in the first place.

It appears amyloid may actually protect delicate brain tissue against inflammation. In fact, amyloid may not be the fire. It may be the smoke. That is, it may be a physiological response to the fire.

This is crucial to understand. If amyloid plaque were not present to buffer against inflammation, then the delicate brain tissues could become damaged. So, for more effective healing, we need to be careful not just to focus on removing the symptoms (the plaque) without addressing the underlying cause.

Here is another example. Patricia had an upper molar that had been mildly painful since she got a crown on it a couple years past. When she finally went to a specialist, he took X-rays of her jaws and maxillary sinuses. He told her there were two issues: one was inflammation around the roots of the tooth, and another was a cyst in her maxillary sinus. He said she needed a root canal, and they would need to monitor the maxillary cyst carefully for the rest of her life.

Patricia, being a student of Eastern medicine, wondered if the maxillary cyst was situated directly above the site of inflammation. The specialist said it was. Patricia hypothesized that the cyst was there to protect the delicate sinus from the inflammation directly below it, at the root of the tooth. She thought that if the inflammation was addressed, the cyst would not be forced to grow or become a problem in itself. She had the tooth pulled, to address the inflammation. There may have been less extreme ways to address it, but it worked. The inflammation resolved. That was over ten years ago, and the maxillary cyst never did become a problem.

It is easy to think the symptom is the problem, when in fact the symptom may be the body's way of handling or minimizing the effect of the root cause. A symptom may arise in response to deeper pathology in the body or mind. It may serve to buffer delicate tissues from the pathology or to generally maintain the status quo. While it is not wrong to address the symptom—the smoke—it *is* possible that if we resolve it without addressing the root cause—the fire—we may cause more damage than good.

Pulses

Prediction isn't limited to predicting the future. There are practical ways we can hone our ability to predict what we will perceive or find in the present. We can assess a patient, predict something we might find, and then check if we are on track.

For example, we can do this every time we take pulses (if that is part of our training). Becoming an adept pulse-reader takes a long time. I'm not sure I know two practitioners who read pulses exactly the same way, and it takes a lot of time working with an adept practitioner to become confident that we know what we are feeling and what it means. But once we learn the basic points of pulse reading, we can teach ourselves to be more adept. We can look at the patient in front of us. We can perceive the visual, audial, and other clues and symptoms, and then predict what we are likely to feel in their pulses *before* we feel them. Then, when we do feel the pulse, if we don't find what we predicted, we ask ourselves, *Why not?* We can then go back to the drawing board and consider what we might have missed that would account for the difference. A patient's pulses should reflect what we see, and vice versa.

Little by little, as we gain confidence in our pulse-reading abilities, we will find that they reflect our predictions more accurately and often. Eventually, the pulses should only serve to refine our predictions and reflections.

I have found some notable exceptions. Once we are generally on-target with pulse predictions, if we find a pulse is radically different than what we expected, it can indicate one of three things. The patient has a history—sometimes a distant history—of intensive exercise; he is taking pharmaceutical or recreational drugs; or he has a very serious pathology. The following are three examples from my practice that illustrate these possibilities. All of them are examples of thin or underweight women with slower pulses than I would expect. I don't recall if there were ever other body types that displayed this kind of discrepancy, but if there were, there were not as many.

Beth was in her 40s, overworked, overstressed, underweight, and very fast talking. I would have expected about 75–80 bpm. Her pulses were 47–52 bpm. My first question when I see pulses slower than I would expect is about exercise. As we probably learned in our medical training, if someone has even a distant history of intensive exercise, it can permanently lower their heart rate. In this case—where the pulse rate did not fit the pattern evidenced in the symptoms—it was important to weight the patient's other symptoms and condition more heavily than her pulse rate. I have found a history of intensive exercise to be a common cause of pulse vs. presentation discrepancy.

Another common reason for this discrepancy is when the patient is taking pharmaceutical or recreational drugs. If they have not reported using these, and do not have a history of intensive exercise, it is worth questioning, if silently, whether they are reporting truthfully or simply omitting that part of their health history. Another common symptom that may accompany use of some prescription drugs is an artificial-looking, pinkish, almost Pepto-Bismol-like hue to the tongue.

Lilly was significantly underweight, spacey, forgetful, and anxiety-ridden. She was convinced she had some disease that was making her dizzy. I fully expected to feel rapid, thin pulses, but they were slow and full. In this case, Lilly was taking pharmaceutical drugs. I've long since forgotten what they were, but they were either for pain or anxiety.

If there is no history of strenuous exercise, and the patient is not currently on medication that may change the nature and qualities of her pulse, there is another, less common possibility.

Barbara was a slight woman with a self-described tendency to anxiety and frustration. It was our first consultation together. According to my perception of Barbara's appearance, sound, traits, and emotions, I expected a wiry, thin, possibly rapid pulse. I was surprised to find it heavy, thick, and of moderate to slow speed.

It turned out that Barbara had cancer she didn't know about. This cancer was lending a slow, thick quality to her pulses that I would not expect to find in a patient with her constitution and main complaints.

Over the years, I have had this experience confirmed on a number of occasions. When there is great discordance between presentation and pulse qualities, but no history of strenuous exercise or current pharmaceutical or recreational drug use, and I do not see the cause for the discrepancy, I find an excuse to gently but firmly refer the patient to a physician I think might be better equipped to do so. In Barbara's case, I could not see the cause of the discrepancy so I referred her to an allopathic physician who was able to diagnose her cancer. If we predict what we will find in the present, and don't find it, it is worth careful review and consideration about why.

The Past: Inferring Past Sexual Relations from the Presence of a Fetus

In this second case, like we infer conception from a pregnancy, we infer past actions or causes by looking at current conditions, consequences, or effects.

A discrepancy between what we see and what a patient says is cause for deeper reflection and more communication. When there is a discrepancy like this, asking more probing questions, with sensitivity, can lead both of us to a greater understanding of the present and the probable cause, or the past. These questions often lead us to interesting places.

A sometimes sensitive example of inferring something in the past from the present is when the patient has a long history of gynecological disorders. This can indicate a history of sexual abuse, even as far past as in childhood.

There is a caveat here, which is that it can sometimes do more damage than good to solicit confirmation of a patient's suspected past. We may infer a history of sexual abuse, but we don't need verbal confirmation of this from our patient. We will treat her gynecological issues the same way in either case, even if sexual abuse is indeed the root cause. If she wishes to disclose this, it may be helpful and lead to even more healing but, in the meantime, we can treat the disorders presented as well as we can, with tenderness and respect. (We will look at this further in Chapter 20.)

There are other clinical examples of current symptoms hinting at curious pasts. It is difficult for me to give examples that I feel certain would apply across the board for CAM practices. I have to turn to my own training and modalities for some examples. Consider this. In Ayurveda, in general, healthy people with sturdy, heavy constitutions tend to have fairly grounded, stable emotions, and those with slight, delicate constitutions tend more to flights of fancy, fear, anxiety, nervous disorders, tics, or twitches. One curious thing I have seen, mostly in women, is this: A patient with all the constitutional and emotional attributes of a delicate constitution is overweight. She is not overeating, under-exercising, or over-stressing—all common causes of weight gain. She is healthy, except she is overweight. When I have seen this, it has not been uncommon for the woman to report or display what some might call "psychic ability." For her, psychic ability might feel commonplace. The extra weight is a benefic response of her body—almost as if the Earth element is rallying to ground her as she follows her ethereal thoughts and experiences. I have seen this often enough that now, when I see this profile, I ask the woman if she feels she has this kind of ability. More often than not she will affirm that she has felt it her entire life. We infer the past from the present situation.

I have seen something similar in men. A strong, sturdy young man, who looks like he could be a boxer, comes to see me. I would not expect a person like this to have any nervous disorders, anxiety, or tics, but he does. There are no obvious stressors in his life, so no apparent cause for his tics or anxiety, and he is not thin. He is not someone I would predict would or should have these symptoms. In cases like these, when the patient and I have talked further, they, too, will admit to having something like psychic abilities or sensitivities. In a man's case, this is a more difficult attribute to fold into his life. For a woman, these abilities are culturally more acceptable than for a big, strong young man who looks like he plays for a sports franchise. This discrepancy between what the young man's culture expects of him and what he knows he is causes him anxiety and results in nervous disorders. To heal these, he will likely have to reach a level of comfort with who he really is.

I am aware that these are odd examples because they really are uncommon, but they each demonstrate that when a patient's presentation is at odds with theory, it is worth looking outside the box and paying extra attention. We have to be sufficiently aware to notice that we are seeing incongruence to begin with, and then carefully infer the current reality based on important factors in the patient's history.

The Future: Inferring Tomorrow's Apple from Today's Apple Seed

This is the culminating form of inference. Once we know there is a fire (that is, we have inferred what is happening in the present from what we are seeing), and we know there must have been sexual relations (that is, we have inferred what happened in the past to have produced what we are seeing in the present), we turn our attention to the future. In this case, we infer future effects, such as an apple, from current causes, like an apple seed. Provided the patient stays on the same course of action, we can plot their likely health trajectory and consider how to reinforce or alter that trajectory, as appropriate.

Rebecca had lost her husband in a terrible car accident and had to work full time to raise three young children on her own. She had, understandably, leaned on some vices to get through those difficult years. She had relied on coffee to get her going in the mornings, processed packaged food for sustenance, an evening drink to help her relax, and cigarettes to help manage the inevitable stress of a life in constant spin.

When she developed nodules on her thyroid, biopsies were inconclusive in determining whether they were malignant or not. When Rebecca inquired about saving half of her thyroid in order to continue getting the benefit of the hormones it secreted, her surgeon strongly urged her to have the entire gland removed. At this point, Rebecca and I had a conversation.

While we both had great respect for this surgeon, and understood the reasoning behind his recommendation, we wanted to consider not just the statistical probability, but what Rebecca's unique trajectory was likely to be. Some months before, as soon as she felt a mass on her thyroid, she had quit drinking, smoking, and using caffeine. She had begun eating whole foods, exercising, and taking steps to reduce the stress in her life. And she was committed to these changes.

We agreed that she probably had a better chance of a positive long-term outcome now than she would have if she had not made those changes. So Rebecca decided to keep half her thyroid. The surgeon reluctantly agreed, but once the pathology reports came back clean on the half of the gland that he had removed, he congratulated Rebecca on her decision.

If Rebecca's previous habits, diet, and lifestyle had contributed to her current condition, her new habits were radically changing her trajectory. If enough of our habits change, and change fast enough, it is sometimes possible to change the outcome in situations like Rebecca's. If her habits had been poor enough, strong enough for long enough, or didn't change, the trajectory could have led toward a poor outcome. Sometimes we don't have sufficient time to make the necessary changes in lifestyle and diet, and we don't have enough time for those changes to shift the momentum of our previous trajectory. While it is easy to quickly change the course of a sailboat, it takes a long time to change the course of an ocean liner. The more severe the problem and the longer it has been present, the longer it is likely to take to turn it around.

Sometimes it is easy for practitioners to confuse their personal projections for thoughtful prediction. We may hope to see something so much that we can be blinded to what is present, but if we can avoid this pitfall, we can help facilitate one of the greatest strengths of Eastern medicine: its focus on preventive medicine. We can consider the patient's weak links, health history, current condition, and the strength of their disorder to infer what will eventually break if they don't change course.

Genetics and Epigenetics

We are entering a time in medicine where genetic testing and results may influence and test our ability to plot a trajectory into the future.

With more and more people getting genetic tests to see if they are predisposed to certain diseases, the question is likely to arise more often, for both patient and doctor: *What do I do with this information?* If, for example, a woman has a gene that predisposes her to a higher risk of breast cancer, what should she do with this information? What should we do?

In this kind of situation, I try not to let fears or seductions govern the thought process or the action. I still try to plot the trajectory. I consider the woman's higher starting risk, and then try to add up any hits that would worsen the situation. For example, alcohol use, stress, smoking, a diet heavy in meat, dairy and highly processed foods, a polluted environment, exposure to endocrine disruptors, and other possible lifestyle or environmental contributors could all be considered "hits." If the woman is a non-drinker, has low stress, eats mostly organic food, lives in a place with clean air, soil and water, and practices other good preventative healthcare practices for her breasts, clearly her risk would be lower. I would consider it very likely that, the more hits she has against her, the greater her risk. Together, she and I would consider her response accordingly. One woman may do well to closely monitor her health and add a few preventative healthcare measures, while a woman with more hits may want to consider more drastic measures, like undergoing a mastectomy.

Genetic risk is real, but so is epigenetic influence. Epigenetics—literally "on top of genetics"—has the potential to trump genetic risk. Epigenetic "tags" sit on top of our genes and activate or deactivate them in response to our experiences and environment. Epigenetic tags turn on genes that prevent disease and turn off genes that cause a variety of illnesses, including breast cancer, heart disease, prostate cancer, and other illnesses. Our diet, stress levels, and exposure to pollutants can all alter our gene expressions.

We are not at the mercy of our genes as much as they are at the mercy of us, at least to some degree.

Here's an example: Dr. Dean Ornish found that more than 500 genes changed course, in response to a vegan diet and lifestyle changes, in only three months.[4] This is due to the influence of the epigenetic tags.

Our bodies—our hormones, organs, tissues and systems, even our genes—do not act in a vacuum. They respond to our environment and thoughts. Environment creates biology. So do thoughts. When we inhale pollutants, our chemistry changes. When we are afraid, our chemistry changes. Conversely, when we enjoy whole food, fresh air, good company, and feed ourselves inspirational thoughts and ideas, we affect our thoughts, emotions, environment, chemistry, epigenetic tags and, ultimately, our genes.

So, when plotting a trajectory—when attempting to infer what the future will hold—we take genetic predisposition into account, but we also take epigenetic influences into account and, in order to do that, we take the positives into account as well as the negatives. We take stock of the "hits" and we take stock of the healthy factors. We can sit with our patients and carefully and honestly assess the story and then support the patient in whatever decision they make. As we sit with them, if we show empathy, we are adding a factor to the positive side.

Reflections

Does inference provide us with knowledge? No. It allows us to guess at the future based on our incomplete knowledge of the present and past, and to try to alter the course of a trajectory.

If we interrupt a negative trajectory so that a patient changes course and *doesn't* get cancer or heart disease, we have no proof that the absence of these diseases was the result of those changes. How do you prove that you averted catastrophe? You can't. But proving is not our job. Doing the best we can, without attachment to the outcome, is the job.

There is so much empirical and researched evidence that lifestyle and diet play a significant part in many chronic and fatal diseases, it would be foolhardy not to strive to interrupt negative trajectories and support positive ones. The combination of learning from authority, cultivating our ability to perceive what is going on, and employing inference allows us to do just that.

How do we make good inferences? How can we build that muscle? In my experience, it comes from having a curiosity about our patients and a hunger for knowledge. We need to be interested in what happened in the past that caused what we are seeing today and in the root of what we are seeing today. This may help us discover the motivating factor at the root of the behavior that led to the current symptoms, and help us navigate a future with greater ease and health.

4 Reflections on Part I

One, the knower of reality, who does not enter into the inner self of the patient with the help of the lamp of knowledge and intelligence, can't treat diseases successfully.
CHARAKA[1]

As we have seen, Charaka writes that we should have excellence in *theoretical* knowledge, and that there are three valid forms of it: authority, perception and inference. When we look into these forms, we find each is imbued with its own particular strengths, vulnerabilities, and distorting influences.

The findings and teachings of studies, professors, and textbooks may be colored by personal, financial, or other bias or motivation. Our senses may be clouded, jaded, or unrefined, thereby coloring what and how we perceive. And our inferences may simply be wrong.

True knowledge, according to Charaka, seems to require the ability to clearly perceive and understand all things the way they were, are, and will be. Who among us can do that? Like the five blind men who each feels a different part of the elephant and describes the whole according to his own limited experience, our knowledge may always be incomplete.

While continuing to pursue knowledge, however, if we can be patient with not knowing, we may find ourselves in the embrace of wisdom. And our example may give our patients a kind of permission to relax into the reality that there is much we can't know. Since stress has been shown conclusively to powerfully influence health, when patients begin to relax, even in the face of illness, isn't this in itself healing?

If it is a bit of a blow to realize how little we know, we may take comfort in this: there are rich rewards for both doctor and patient from even the pursuit of knowledge.

The following are the happy side effects of the pursuit of knowledge.

Humility

The secret of humility is that we have
something to learn from everyone.
KIRPAL SINGH

Humility does not consist in hiding our talents and virtues,
in thinking ourselves worse and more ordinary than we
are, but in possessing a clear knowledge of all that is
lacking in us, and not exalting ourselves for that which we
have, seeing that God has freely given it us, and with all
His gifts, we are still infinitely of little importance.
JEAN-BAPTISTE HENRI LACORDAIRE

This Lacordaire quote may be one of my favorites. If we truly strive for knowledge, we cannot help but come to the conclusion that most of us truly know very little. If humility is simply an honest and accurate understanding of our limitations, it is a healthy side effect of the honest pursuit of knowledge.

Humility differs from insecurity. Being clear and honest about our limitations is not a display of weakness. It is a strength, as it keeps us open, curious about what we can learn from our patients, and vigilant as to what may best help facilitate their healing.

Confidence

Paradoxically, as we pursue theoretical knowledge—even knowing its limitations—we may find our confidence grows.

Though knowledge itself is dispassionate and relentless, aloof from and unconcerned with our beliefs or confidences, the act of pursuing knowledge may strengthen our beliefs and confidence, such as confidence in a herb or remedy. We can't help it. As we listen to a professor, read a new study, or find our ability to perceive or infer is growing more accurate, we gain inspiration and confidence.

The pursuit of knowledge, then, begets confidence as well as humility—unlikely bedfellows, but possibly a perfect coupling when it comes to character and a beneficial approach with patients, because patients trust confident—but not arrogant—doctors.

Communication, Empathy, Improved Diagnosis and Outcomes

When, in the pursuit of knowledge, we work to refine our sensory abilities, there is a cascade of positive effects. We gain more empathy and become better able to communicate effectively with our patients. As a result, our ability to diagnose improves, as does the trust between our patients and ourselves. With increased trust comes increased compliance, and a better chance of a positive clinical outcome.[2]

The Tally

The pursuit of knowledge itself, then, yields at least six positive side effects: humility, confidence, improved communication skills, empathy, improved accuracy in diagnosis, and better treatment outcomes for our patients. If we were going to compile a list of defining characteristics of someone who embodies the art of medicine, wouldn't those first five side effects be near the top?

This means that although we may be unable to benefit our patients with our knowledge, incomplete as it is, they will benefit simply from our *pursuit* of knowledge.

If we consistently and concurrently persist in the quest for knowledge, and remain mindful of how little we actually do know, we may join the ranks of a humble and humbling profession.

PART II

Extensive Practical Experience

Things We May Not Learn in School

*Learning, wisdom, practical knowledge, experience,
accomplishment, and popularity—of these, even one quality
is sufficient to lend significance to the title of physician.
One who possesses all auspicious qualities like learning,
etc., deserves to hold the honorable degree of physician—
one who showers happiness on the living beings.*
CHARAKA[1]

A degree is only the beginning of an education. As much as we may gain and earn humility, confidence, improved communication skills, empathy, and improved accuracy in diagnosis in the quest for knowledge, experience can further refine each of these attributes that are so central to the art of medicine. You will have had your own experiences. Here are a few things I've learned through mine. This is not a comprehensive list of things we should all know. They are random things I was not taught in school and couldn't find in books; things I learned along the way. If I were to revisit these issues in ten years' time, I expect my perspective on some of them would change.

In our training, we learn diagnostic techniques and theories, and we learn technical applications and skills. To learn how to apply this theoretical knowledge elegantly to living patients requires more than memorization. It requires the light of clarity gained though our own experience. And it sometimes requires stumbling along—sometimes quite badly—until we can reach, if not elegance, at least some degree of understanding.

5 Don't Panic. Wait.

*Take ten steps in the dark with a lantern and
the next ten steps will be revealed.*
BUDDHA

With the awareness of how little we really know sometimes, it could be easy to panic.

Don't.

Things work out anyway.

There have been so very many times when I sat with a patient, began to hear their story, and started to panic. *Oh no. I'm not going to know what to do, say, or prescribe! I don't know how to fix this!* In these moments, the best thing I have found to do is not panic. To breathe deeply, relax, let go of any agenda I might have—including to "fix" anything, practice what I have learned about really seeing, really hearing, and really feeling what is happening, and trust that something will become clear.

However complicated the patient's symptoms or history, however dire or overwhelming the moment feels, however puny or insufficient my own understanding, experience, or training seems, if I take a breath and remember to align with That-Which-Is-Bigger-Than-Me, something becomes clear. It always has. Maybe this clarity is a knowing, after all.

Sometimes people talk about alchemy in relation to the healing process. To me, alchemy has come to mean this: we can go so far into reality that we transform. Which makes it seem like reality itself is transforming. And maybe it is. When we surrender deeply to not knowing, something becomes known to us. We surrender to discomfort, and comfort rises, like the phoenix from the ashes. We surrender to confusion and clarity dawns. In my experience, this clarity often dawns simultaneously in both the patient and the doctor. It is an intimate experience, as if we have both been visited by Truth, Rightness, and Goodness. We both feel something has already changed. It is often the case that the patient will experience a deep knowing about what is needed. Sometimes I am visited with a knowing. It's as if a path that was covered in debris is cleared off. Maybe we can't see the end of the path yet, but we can see the next step.

If I am patient and sacrifice my will, ideas, decisions, and desire to fix things, I relax, the patient senses this and relaxes, and transformation happens. We might wait in silence for a bit, and this silence can be a place of refuge, transformation, and possibility. There can even be comfort in the uncertainty. We both are willing to go someplace new and explore the mystery. And the next step becomes clear.

What I'm describing may sound lofty and esoteric, but if you have ever experienced this, either as a patient or a doctor, you will recognize it. It is hard to describe, but when we wade into the mystery, transformation happens. Our inner knowing becomes known. And the patient carries that with them when they leave our office.

Sometimes it takes more courage to wait than to do something. When things are unclear, wait. Something always changes.

6 Nothing Is Ever as It Seems

Or, at least, nothing is ever *only* as it seems.

There is an old story about a master who asks his disciple to go to the village, purchase some flour, and bring it back to him. His disciple does as she is asked, but doesn't notice that the bag of flour, which she is carrying on her shoulder, has a hole in it. All the way back to her master's, the flour slowly pours out of the hole. Upon her return, she realizes what has happened. She is mortified. She didn't see the hole. She is so sorry. She begs his forgiveness. But the master says, "Don't worry. You did exactly as I asked. I knew this would happen, and it is the very reason I asked you to do this. You see, I wanted a clearly marked path from here to the village."

Like the woman, we think we know what we are about, what we are doing, and what we are diagnosing, treating, and healing. But it may be that the most good we do is through actions, gestures, conversations, or experiences that we don't even remember. Maybe it is enough to show up in integrity.

My guru used to say that a bird doesn't fly over your head without your having that much destiny with that bird. I learned from him that if we have the destiny to meet with someone as our patient, we cannot keep them away, no matter how hard we try. And if we don't, we cannot bring them to us as a patient, no matter how hard we try.

Certainly we want to do the best we can, with the knowledge we have, to facilitate maximum healing, but that is most likely to happen when our primary practice is to be in integrity, in an undivided state of wholeness, ready to meet our destiny with this person.

7 Doctor as Educator

No doctor since the beginning of time has ever cured a
patient. No doctor ever will, for Nature alone can cure.
Physicians are not meant to work wonders or perform
miracles. A true physician is a teacher who helps his or
her patients work through their problems at all levels.
DR. ROBERT E. SVOBODA[1]

Dr. Ngawang Chopel, a Nepali *vaidya* (traditionally trained Ayurvedic practitioner), is said to have declared, "The shepherd picks up his lunch bag and goes to heaven. The doctor picks up his medicine bag and goes to hell."[2]

When I first read this, I submitted my own silent "Amen!" What he actually meant, I don't remember and can't say, but what it means to me is this: the shepherd is responsible for keeping his sheep alive, protected, fed, and accounted for. He is serving them and shall be rewarded for it. He is not giving them advice for which he will be held accountable. But this is not often the case with physicians, who can spend their professional lives dispensing advice, whether to eat or avoid certain foods, activities, or relationships, to ingest certain medicines, or to adhere to some remedial regime.

According to the law of karma—or perhaps simple understanding—it would follow that the physician would shoulder some responsibility for the outcome when someone takes his advice. I have also been told by wise people in my life that the physician shares in the fruit of the actions that their patients go on to create, once they are healed. These is weighty stuff indeed—stuff I personally like to keep to a minimum, knowing my shoulders are not that broad nor my constitution that sturdy.

As an extreme example, if a murderer comes to the doctor and is suffering from great pain, pain that prevents him from committing more murders, and the doctor assists him—relieving him of his pain, thus enabling him to commit more murders—does the doctor share in the responsibility for those crimes? Should the physician be blind to who "deserves" to be treated and simply do his best to provide relief to all, without discrimination? Or is the doctor obliged to withhold treatment from people who intend to harm others? It is rare to encounter such dire examples, but similar, though far less extreme, situations occur with each patient we treat. Human and karmic complications, implications, and ramifications may be beyond our capacity to fully understand, but it doesn't mean they are not valid considerations.

I remember attending a circus cabaret show. At the beginning of the show, the emcee commanded, "Leave your troubles and worries at the door. You are in our hands now!" I remember thinking how courageous that was: to willingly invite the responsibility for other human beings. For myself, in practice, issuing such an invitation would have to be the result of ignorance, courage, or irrepressible love, like that of a parent for a child.

It feels weighty to extend an invitation to someone to put themselves in our hands. Another option, for the meeker of us, is to explain treatment options, convey information, and perhaps share what we might do or have done if or when we were in our patient's shoes. Then we leave the final decision up to them about whether or not to take a medication, make a change in diet, have a treatment, or change their life in some way. After all, no matter what my previous experience or what I may have learned, I do not know the ramifications that will occur once someone has chosen to tread a certain path. Nor am I aware how much responsibility for these ramifications is ultimately on my shoulders. These considerations feed my preference for education over prescription.

Perhaps education has always been part of the job. The word "doctor" is derived from the Latin word for "teacher." Of course, there are times when the last thing a patient wants to do, or can do, is make his own medical decisions. If this is truly the case, a family member may need to make the decision. Either way, I have found that an honest discussion of the possible courses of actions and outcomes yields a fairly clear course of action. This way, it often feels like my patient or her family and I are arriving at a conclusion together.

While it may be ethically or karmically tricky business to provide advice to patients about their physical health, my guru taught me that it is all the more weighty and tricky to dispense spiritual prescriptions. He clearly discouraged his disciples, including me, from dispensing spiritual directions, suggestions, *mantras*, prayers, or spiritual techniques to anyone, lest we risk becoming responsible for the spiritual welfare of another. He counseled that unless we fully know what that entails, and have the direct order to do so from someone who in turn incurs responsibility for what we do, it is much too weighty a responsibility for most of us to bear.

I cannot fathom the complicated reality of karmas, nor can I foresee the ramifications of all my actions. So I endeavor to do the best I can in any particular case with what I am given to know and feel, to ask my guru to protect both the patient and me, and to leave the results to the Divine.

Not telling people what to do not only saves us from the obvious or subtle consequences involved, but it can serve to empower the patient to participate consciously in her own physical or spiritual healthcare, and consider for herself whether the medicine or *mantra* is working. If we dictate what she is doing, it is more likely that her own awareness will lay dormant, and it will then be our job to assess what is working and how, instead of hers.

Finally, working with patients as partners in their healthcare, instead of directing them to do or change certain things, supports a dynamic of equality and collaboration rather than hierarchy. It helps us both to align our views of their past and present health situation, and to forge together a good direction for the future.

8 Treat Complicated with Simple

The new practitioner has 100 different treatments for each patient who walks through the door. The experienced practitioner has one treatment for 100 patients who walk through the door.
ANONYMOUS CHINESE MEDICINE APHORISM

This is one of my all-time favorite quotes regarding medicine.

I have found it to be true across the board. Over and over and over. Whether or not a patient presents with migraine, gynecological issues, chronic conditions, anxiety, or a myriad of other disorders, the root causes of all these disorders often lie in the basic foundations of life: lifestyle, diet, or emotional stress. The results simply manifest differently in different people, depending on their unique challenges. Whatever the particular disorder, if we address the basic foundations of life and the patient chooses to attend to these areas, many disorders may lessen or resolve entirely on their own.

Addressing all three aspects of the triad of lifestyle, diet, and stress is essential. Can you focus on diet to the exclusion of lifestyle? Can you erase the effects of a bad diet by having a good exercise routine? Generally not. All components work together to create a healthy, solid foundation.

Since we need to address all three aspects with most patients, we may find ourselves repeating information and prescriptions over and over. This isn't a unique problem. When I was writing *Balance Your Hormones, Balance Your Life*, I found it hard not to be overly repetitive.

When we look at what we can do to prevent breast cancer, osteoporosis, heart disease, or just about any other women's health ailment covered in that book, we find we need to address lifestyle, diet, and stress levels, along with any other specific additional measures. That can make for a lot of repetition. In *The China Study*, the authors found a similar problem. They wrote that their editor "asked, in effect, 'can you make specific diet plans for each disease, so that every chapter doesn't have the same recommendations?'" But they couldn't deliver that. They wrote that they didn't "have a different, catchy formula for each disease."[1] Certain dietary patterns benefited all the diseases. Repetition may not be exciting. It may not be impressive. Editors might not like it. It may not boost our egos. It may even be a little embarrassing. Plus, if we are trained in medical systems that pride themselves on treating each person as a unique individual, we may be tempted to prescribe very differently to each person.

While each person is indeed unique, the foundational concerns are important for everyone, and addressing them may lessen or resolve root problems in a way that no herb or remedy can. No matter the size or shape of the building, a strong foundation is always important. Renowned martial artist Bruce Lee said, "I fear not the man who has practiced 10,000 kicks once, but I fear the man who has practiced one kick 10,000 times." Becoming adept at supporting these basic concerns can make the difference between offering temporary relief and supporting permanent, effective healing.

One of the seriously intimidating situations for new practitioners is when a patient presents with a very complicated, lengthy health history, a long list of pharmaceutical drugs or supplements that they are committed to, and a list of odd reactions they have had to various substances.

In cases like this, there is a tendency to try to meet complicated with complicated. We are tempted to throw out the "one size fits most" approach of addressing the basic components of lifestyle and diet considerations, and try to address each symptom. We create or prescribe a complicated protocol, complete with a herb mix with a long list of ingredients or many different remedies, in order to address each of the patient's complaints and conditions. But in these cases, it may be more important than ever, and often more effective, to stay committed to simple.

One serious problem with treating complicated cases with complicated protocols and formulas is that the more supplements or medications a patient is taking, the higher the likelihood of complications with, or distressing side effects from, any treatment, including herbs and remedies. There is a fundamental tenet of many medical modalities: treat symptoms and diseases with substances that possess opposite qualities.

For example, if a disease is hot, we employ the cold quality to counteract it. If it is a problem of heaviness, we want to employ the light quality. If it is dry, we lubricate it, and so on. By the same principle, if something is complicated, we would want to treat it with simple. Introduce more simplicity into the person's life, routines, and remedies (if we prescribe any) to counteract the complexity of their lives and the complicated nature of their disorders. In these cases, if any remedy is given, the simpler the better. One-ingredient formulas may be especially prudent. Then we can watch, wait, and consider the effects of this single ingredient before adding anything else.

Keeping things simple may also benefit many patients by antidoting the complicated nature of the world in which we live and the influences to which we are exposed. Even if we try to source our goods and food locally, for example, most of us live in dwellings constructed from materials sourced globally. At least some of our food, drinks, spices, and clothes come from distant countries, and the vast majority of us are under the influence of globally sourced thoughts, ideas, and memes. We are controlling our environments *and* being controlled by them. It is too complicated, too messy, too powerful, and too stimulating to figure out.

The myriad vectorial influences that contribute to the mental, spiritual, emotional, and physical conditions of our patients are too numerous and nuanced for most of us to be able to identify and either counteract or amplify as needed. Most of us simply do not possess that level of sophisticated awareness.

When we address the context of the patient's life, exploring ways to simplify it, before adding any more complications into the mix, it is safer for patients and allows time for at least some of the complicated symptoms to abate without introducing complicated medicines.

When the waves are choppy, chaotic, erratic, and buffeting, we can put on our diving gear and dive under the surface to reach a deep, still place. The more complicated the picture looks, the quieter we can become, and the more deeply we can look, listen, and feel. Something will become clear. And sometimes things will become simple.

A possibility may occur to us, one we had not previously seen. New perspectives and possibilities arise when we let go and quietly wait.

Certainly there can be exceptions to this. Complicated cases may occasionally require complicated strategies or treatment to address them effectively but, usually, going back to the vitally important foundational points is an imperative and effective starting point. This can be especially important to keep in mind with patients with a history of odd responses or reactions to many substances or medicines. (We'll explore that later, in Chapter 30.)

The question may arise—if we treat complicated with simple, should we treat simple with complicated? And the answer might be, "Yes." For example, if someone is in good health and already has a healthy diet and lifestyle and low stress, they may be good candidates for experimentation. They have a strong enough foundation to clearly see how what they do affects them. They can better assess the effects of their actions and the food or substances they ingest, so they could experiment with intricate or complicated physical, mental, or breathing exercises, or the use of herbal substances.

Remember, we don't have to do everything at once. We just have to do something. If we wait for that something to become clear, if we don't rush it, it will make itself known. Together, the patient and doctor can take a step…and wait.

9 The Power of Subtraction

When we are troubleshooting lifestyle, diet, and stress, it is often helpful to employ medicine of subtraction before adding anything else to a patient's life and to-do list.

Here's what happens. We are addicted to foods or other substances of poor quality or quantity, or use them with poor timing. As a result, our digestive systems and organs are taxed, and low-grade malaise or illness follows. We feel poorly, so we consume more substances—this time in the form of medicines to make ourselves feel better. This approach has limitations and ramifications.

First, when our digestive capacity is compromised, it is not strong enough even to digest food efficiently, much less to cope with the morbidity present in the digestive system due to illness, *and* process the medicine we are taking for it, all at the same time. If we can't digest our medicine, it may be of less—if any—value, and we run the risk of further complicating or weakening our digestive strength or our disorders.

Second, so many of the medicinal herbs we have used in Eastern medicine have been over-harvested and are not being grown in a sustainable way. As a result, many have become rare or endangered and risk extinction.

If we can find a way to support our patients without prescribing herbs, we are extracting less of a toll on the earth as well as our patients' pocketbooks.

The first step (or at least a concurrent one) in any treatment plan for a chronic problem might be to support our patients more enthusiastically to once and for all reduce or quit the intake of substances that are causing them harm—including poor quality or quantity of food—and to counsel them or refer them to counseling for addiction. (We'll look at this later.) Either after this subtraction is successful, or concurrently—depending on the patient and circumstances—we can offer education on good quality food and healthy lifestyle changes, including appropriate exercise and stress reduction techniques. Then we wait. Maybe a month. Maybe six. And we see what remains. Often, if the person truly makes those changes, many of their health problems will fall away, leaving perhaps only one or two stubborn challenge areas. These may require tailored herbs or other remedies—medicines of addition—to manage or cure them.

This method not only protects the digestive strength of our patients and the bounty of the earth; it also protects our patients' finances, as it is cheaper to subtract substances than to add them.

So, first comes the medicine of subtraction: get rid of the poisons in life—the poisonous addictions, foods, experiences, pastimes, jobs, and thoughts.

Then wait. Then add herbs and remedies, if needed.

Naturally there are times when it is important to prescribe herbs or remedies immediately, before there is time for lifestyle and diet changes to take effect, but "subtraction before addition" is a general strategy to keep in mind.

10 Patients Should Get Better

I have not failed. I've just found 10,000 ways that won't work.
THOMAS A. EDISON

Patients should get better.

Well, yes and no.

My husband, Jim Ventresca, a doctor of Oriental Medicine, treated an elderly woman with acupuncture for her back pain for some months with little effect on the pain. When he said, "Elyse, I don't think your pain is responding to acupuncture," she exclaimed, "Oh no, Doctor! Does that mean I have to stop coming for treatment?!" She had been feeling benefit from the relationship and feeling better overall from the acupuncture, even if her back pain was not improving.

Voltaire is widely attributed to have said, "The art of medicine consists in amusing the patient while nature cures the disease." While this may be an oversimplification or not always true, there can certainly be something sustaining and comforting about the doctor–patient relationship that can carry the patient through the time it takes for a problem to heal (or not), whether it heals on its own or in response to a medicine or therapy or whether it never heals at all.

Any physician in practice long enough is aware that there are patients who either do not get better, or at least do not get better in some areas. And, at some point, the natural conclusion of a condition is death. In Ayurveda, there are four categories of illness: that which can be easily treated and cured; that which that can be cured with difficulty; that which, while incurable, is manageable; and that which is neither manageable nor curable.[1]

Not all patients will "get better," at least in terms of a targeted disease. But as long as there is breath, there is hope for some aspect of improvement in the patient. Even as a patient lies dying, there may be ways to support his comfort and peace of mind—perhaps something as simple as sitting quietly and offering a reassuring presence. Patients should get better in some way: feel more comforted, experience less pain, or be cured.

With elderly or very ill patients with one or more organs failing, curing medical conditions may well not be their primary concern. Our focus at that point may be to learn what their goals are for their health and lives and how we can support them. Maybe looking at creative ways to help them improve balance and avoid falling. Maybe sitting with the family to go over an advanced directive form.

In CAM, practitioners will often feel satisfied with there being an overall benefit, even if there is little or no benefit to the original medical complaint. As my friend and colleague, Edward Kentish, L.Ac., points out, "Everybody needs a ticket in the door. We're in relationship-based healing." He suggests—and this is a common sentiment and practice in CAM—that it takes time for pathology to unravel—first to reveal its complexity and then to heal, layer by layer. It is not so much about the "shoulder pain" that brings a patient in the door, as it is about the patient's wellbeing as a whole.

I find this to be quite true, but I have also found it is easy to fall into apathy unawares—to submit to the momentum of a certain treatment strategy, once established, and forget to remain vigilant as to whether the strategy continues to be the best one as time progresses. We sometimes forget to question why a patient is not improving, or to take the time to recognize that a patient no longer wishes to focus on treating a medical condition and would prefer to start focusing on their quality of life for its remainder. When we fail to pay attention to these shifting realities, we are robbed of the option to shift to a more effective plan, if possible, or to re-commit to the originally chosen path.

I had a patient who was a practicing nurse. When Lisa first came in, her pulses were relaxed, but her Liver energy was strained. I saw Lisa for at least 25 patient visits for acupuncture. Throughout this time she reported eating well, exercising appropriately, and experiencing no undue stress. In fact, she seemed quite relaxed, especially for her constitution (very thin and wiry) and age (late 40s), which often indicate a constitution and age that tends to higher anxiety. Despite her apparently good habits and disposition, and the fact that she always reported feeling good after her acupuncture treatments, Lisa's Liver pulse continued to be weak. Nothing she reported seemed to account for the fact that there was no improvement.

I didn't think much of it at the time. I was in the momentum we had created together—we were both satisfied with her overall sense of enhanced wellbeing—and I did not question why her Liver pulses remained as weak as they had been at her first appointment. I assumed her Liver weakness was either in the "manageable but not curable" category of disease or the "curable with difficulty" category, perhaps due to a past history of stress or substance abuse. But I was also lulled into personal satisfaction, in part because of Lisa's satisfaction. In any case, somewhere along the line I stopped being concerned about her Liver pulse.

One day Lisa did not show up for her appointment. The next time I saw one of her colleagues, I learned Lisa had been addicted to painkillers, was caught forging her own prescriptions, and had been fired. She had dropped out of her normal social circles. I never saw or heard from Lisa again. Maybe she was too embarrassed to return. Maybe she could no longer afford treatment. Maybe something else was going on for her. In any case, I was moved to consider how I could have missed something so big for so long.

Lisa and I had had a good rapport, and I had trusted she would share all the important factors about her health. I had not worked with many people addicted to pills and was not vigilant about this possibility. Not all healthcare providers have much experience with addicts and addictions. We need to keep in mind that addiction is always a possible factor, and it may be more common than we expect. (We'll talk more about addiction later.) We especially need to consider whether addiction could be a factor if our patient is not improving, even after altering important lifestyle and dietary factors, and taking herbs and other remedies or treatments.

Perhaps even with more experience I would have missed Lisa's addiction; addicts are often practiced at hiding their addictions.

But it was a good lesson for me to dig deeper, to consistently look for what is not obvious, for what I might be missing. Lisa's job did give her easy access to pills, but anyone in any job can be addicted to something, no matter their race, religion, profession, financial position, or social class. If a patient is not improving, addiction is a possible cause.

How could I have discovered the truth in Lisa's situation? It may or may not have been possible, but this is what I would do differently now: I would consider that women of her constitution, age, and life circumstances often suffer from anxiety, so I would dig into this more. Why were her pulses relaxed even though her Liver pulse was weak? (Usually, if the Liver pulse is weak, the overall pulse has more tension to it.) She had a job many would find stressful. What was she doing to counteract that stress? Had she logged considerable time learning or practicing meditation, yoga, or some other spiritual practice or perspective? In Lisa's case, the answer was no, and I would have paid more attention to that and considered what might be keeping her on such an even keel in her life. And I would have taken note of her access to drugs.

It's true that many patients don't get better in every way. But it is good to avoid the understandable momentum towards becoming apathetic or robotic in our treatment. It is good to remain alert to reasons why the patient is not improving, and be conscientious in searching for other ways to help them heal.

When we become complacent, we can miss things. There is a big difference between accepting God's will and being complacent. It is our job to continue to make the efforts. The results are not in our hands. We accept that—and we continue making our best efforts.

Theologian Fredrick Buechner wrote: "It is absolutely crucial... to keep in constant touch with what is going on in your own life's story and to pay close attention to what is going on in the stories of others' lives. If God is present anywhere, it is in those stories that God is present."[2]

My guru taught me that no medicine works without the presence of God in it, and that attention, being a representative of consciousness, is a link to God, the Ocean of consciousness. When we are paying attention, then we are consciously or otherwise bringing an element of awareness and divinity to medicine.

11 When Nothing Is Wrong, Pay Close Attention

Of course, we always want to pay close attention, but it is easy to think that this is not necessary when a patient presents no major complaints, has a blank health history intake, and reports no problems. But there is a reason she scheduled a healthcare visit, and we may need to pay close attention to tease out what that reason is.

I mentioned earlier that my guru used to say that a bird doesn't fly over your head without your having that much destiny with it. I used to think about this in my practice, and resolved to believe that, whatever else appeared to be happening, it was certain that I had some karma (what my guru sometimes called "give and take") with that person. Whether or not the patient has a major health concern, he has scheduled an appointment and shown up for a reason. The best way to honor that connection is for me to listen closely to the issues and feelings that arise in these meetings—not only from my patient, but from myself—and address them with as much integrity and care as I can. When the connection is done, the patient moves on.

A 50-year-old patient came to see me with only one complaint. He had some pain in his small toe. The rest of his intake form was blank. Upon talking with him further, I learned that he had been born female and had recently undergone operations and had drug therapy to become male. He was very much at peace with his decision, as was his partner, but he needed some support in what was not yet a complete transition. To be able to listen and provide simple acupuncture and a non-judgmental safe place was enough. It was our relationship, as much as any remedy, that supported this patient's health.

12

Healing Through Environment, Co-Workers, and Protocols

(This Is Not as Boring as It Sounds)

Environment

I recently received a letter from a young man who is very dear to me. He wrote that although nature heals, he appreciated the importance of "the conditions in which nature can work its magic."

In this day and age, where the busy are glorified and the relaxed mocked, maintaining a peaceful presence may not be de rigueur—it can even feel awkward at times, either for the physician or the patient—but it may be essential to counteract the frenetic pace of life afflicting many patients today. In the same way that we treat complicated with simple, we can treat frenetic with calm.

If neutral and peaceful conditions are created in our waiting rooms and treatment rooms—and cultivated by our employees and associates—our patients may begin to improve before we ever see them. Their stress may melt, at least in part, and they may be more receptive to healing and change.

I sometimes spend time at Vaidyagrama, an Ayurvedic "eco-village" outside of Coimbatore, India, where there are no sound systems, alcohol, junk food, or drugs, and little in the way of internet accessibility. None of the patients or guests here are ever nagged to eat good food, avoid mind-altering substances, limit their screen time, or get enough rest. There is no need. The environment does the whole job. Only healthy food is available. The other stuff isn't.

This is a concept that has been employed in healthcare for centuries. Consider the history of sanitariums.

In sanitariums, clean food, clean water, and especially clean air were considered essential elements for health. These places were usually comfortable, sometimes luxurious resorts located in pristine natural settings. To nurse guests back to robust health, they were exposed to high altitude, fresh air, and good nutrition, and were expected to adopt healthy daily routines that included an early bedtime.

Russian sanitariums, like the Ayurvedic eco-village, are still deliberately designed to make the best use of the natural environment. Guests' lodging may be located half a kilometer from where meals are served, and one kilometer from the waters, so they are forced to walk and breathe fresh air over the course of their daily activities.

I had the opportunity to speak with Konstantin Leonidovich Popov, educated as a paramedic and nurse cum masseur, with four years of medical school. He worked as a massage therapist from 2005–2008 at "Tes,"[1] which is short (in Russian) for something warm and fuzzy like, "Regional Government Autonomous Institution, Central Complex of Social Services." It is one of the oldest, most established sanitariums in Russia. Like many of the Russian sanitariums, Tes is located in a rural place of beauty, in the middle of the forest, and is rich in the essential ingredients of fresh air, water, and food.

Popov told me that most people benefit enormously from their time at the sanitarium—not surprising given that, like Popov, all healthcare practitioners at Russian sanitariums are highly trained professionals. Guests begin their stay by being evaluated by a team of physicians and undergoing any necessary tests. They are then subject to a rigorous treatment regimen.

I asked Popov whether he thought the success of the sanitariums and the health benefits to their guests were due to the treatments from the highly trained staff, or simply a result of spending time in a beautiful natural environment. Without hesitation, Popov replied that he felt that most of the good effects were due to the environment.

Whether we have a sanitarium on many acres of land or one small treatment room, we can consider using all five senses to help encourage health.

We can have fresh, clean air—not scented, since many patients are sensitive to even 100 percent natural incense or essential oils. When there are no strong scents, there is less stimulation or association that may trigger emotional or physical responses. In my office, we kept all aromatic foods and drinks out of the building, and everyone who worked there avoided wearing scents of any kind. We also had houseplants in our office, as they both clean the air and are visually appealing.

We can also appeal to the visual sense with neutral, beautiful artwork or statues or paint jobs unlikely to alienate anyone with any particular religious belief, including atheism.

We can appeal to the sense of taste by having water or herbal teas available.

We can have calming music playing or simple silence to counteract or soothe the audial bombardment many of us are habituated to. At least since the time of the Great Yellow Emperor in China (2698–2598 BCE), it has been believed in China that music can heal, stabilize, and strengthen the body, soul, character, and conduct. The pentatonic scale relates to the five elements of Chinese Medicine, and correlates with five important internal organs and the five sensory organs: the eyes, ears, skin, mouth, and nose. One of the earliest purposes of music in China was to heal. In fact, the Chinese character for medicine comes from the character for music.[2]

Finally, we can work with tactile experience to support a sense of stability. This is one sense we may not often consider, but it can be influential. Touch is the first sense we develop. We have used our hands since we were born to acquire information about our environments. Indeed, haptically acquired information creates a scaffold for how we feel about the world around us, what judgments we make, and how we communicate.

Experiments have shown that tactile sensations from heavy or light, smooth or rough, and soft or hard objects unconsciously influence our impressions, judgments, decisions, and interactions. They also affect how strict or flexible we are—or perceive others to be. When we hold a heavy clipboard, for example, we are more likely to view a situation as grave or important than if we are holding a light object.[3] This works both ways. If we think an object is important, we tend to estimate that it is physically heavier than if we think it is of trivial importance.[4] Our tactile perceptions influence our experience.

Feeling surfaces and objects that are hard tends to produce perceptions of strictness, rigidity, and stability, and may increase our own or our patient's tendency to act this way in our communications. While strict and rigid may not be what we are going for, stability can indeed be a valuable message. It is not that any of these qualities are inherently good or bad. They are simply there, have an effect, and we can consider that effect when designing our treatment and waiting rooms.

The field of "embodied cognition" has studied how qualities in our environment affect our perception and experience of the world, and it turns out, and as Eastern medicine teaches, like increases like.

It may not come as a surprise to practitioners familiar with this concept, that our emotions affect our experience of physical phenomenon and vice versa. For example, when we feel socially isolated or excluded, we feel that a room is colder than we think it is when we feel included. An "icy" stare from someone can affect our subjective experience of temperature, making us crave physical as well as emotional warmth.[5]

This works both ways. The temperature of a room or a drink may affect how we perceive the warmth of people we interact with, and have an impact on how much we open up to them, or they to us. For example, a study published in the journal *Science* in 2008 demonstrated that qualities like heat and cold affect our emotional as well as physical wellbeing. When people evaluated the effect of a heating pad or held a warm beverage for ten to fifteen seconds, they were more likely to open up and "warm" to strangers. They were even more likely to perceive the strangers as warm individuals than were test subjects who evaluated the effect of a cold pack or held a cold drink. This second group perceived the opposite effect.[6]

Because our patients' and our own first impressions and sensory experiences are liable to be influenced by our five senses, controlling our environment is worth considering. If our office, waiting room, treatment room, employees, and we ourselves strive towards warmth and sensory neutrality, the healing process can be enhanced.

We could put this idea to more specific use and have two treatment rooms, for example: one that has many soft, smooth, heavy things and calming music in order to promote these qualities, and another that has more light-hearted music, more stimulating artwork, and brighter lights for patients who need to be more stimulated. (The latter may not be as much in demand in a world that is already over-stimulated.) In my office, we opted for a balance of these sets of opposites. For example, we had sturdy chairs that had give in them, and soft treatment tables. We kept all rooms warm enough that patients could change into dressing gowns without feeling chilled. There were always hot and cool drinks available.

If we are working within a medical modality that recognizes five elements, we could even have five treatment rooms, one dedicated to each of the elements, complete with associated music, color, shapes, and other sensory ingredients.

We could go further and employ principles of Feng Shui, *vastu shastra*, or other forms of geomancy. Vaidyagrama—the Ayurvedic eco village—did just that. Its builders adhered so closely to the principles of *vastu shastra* that they tore down and rebuilt a wall that was only a handful of centimeters off from the ideal dimensions. We may not be able to easily measure the effects of this dedication on the patients at Vaidyagrama, but we can consider for ourselves how our environment affects us.

Co-Workers

Having receptionists and office managers, and working with associates, can be wonderful. It can help us work more efficiently and help our patients feel, and indeed be, more supported. But it can also be scary. I have friends who have been in practice for years and could probably use the help, but who are afraid to hire anyone, for fear the new person may alter the experience in their office.

If we consider closely what is important to us and are clear about it with our co-workers, we can maintain or enhance the neutral, healing environment we are working to provide.

When I hired office managers, or considered bringing in associates, we would have a conversation about providing a neutral, welcoming space. If they were comfortable with conversing and spending time with anyone, regardless of sex, race, sexual orientation, age, class, or political leaning, and if they were willing to keep aromatic food and drinks—including coffee—out of the building, they were likely to be a good fit. Generally I found people understood that many patients are trying to reduce or quit drinking coffee, sugary drinks, or processed food, and that it was most supportive to keep those things out of the office.

It is also important that employees do not give patients medical advice, especially as the patient may well feel that this advice is sanctioned by the physician and do as suggested. This advice may not be in line with what you would recommend. In addition, we can be legally responsible for things our employees do and say to our patients.

Here is the information I used to give to anyone who was going to work in my office:

Every employer has their idiosyncrasies. I'd like you to know mine up front.

This is a place of healing, and the experience I wish for people is that of total health. This means different things for different people, so these guidelines are designed to create a neutral environment so that most everyone seeking health feels comfortable. Some of the following restrictions may seem tedious, but they are important to me and to many of my patients.

- Maintain an attitude of welcome and genuine appreciation for all patients and visitors, regardless of gender, religious beliefs, sexual orientation, political ideology, general belief systems, etc. This is the most important point.

- No food in the building. (Snacks that are not messy—crumbs, sticky, juicy, and the like—have no odor, are kept out of sight, and are not consumed in front of patients or while on the phone are okay. Food crumbs invite cockroaches, and if a patient is changing into a gown and sees a roach, it kind of changes the experience for them. So far I've never seen a cockroach in the building.)

- No coffee in the building. While I love the smell, some of my patients are trying to quit coffee, and the aroma is pervasive.

- No non-vegetarian food on the premises (including on the porch area or driveway, unless it is in your car).

- Any soft drinks, sugary drinks, etc., drunk on the premises should be in a personal cup rather than a can or juice-box, out of consideration for patients trying to cut down on sugar.

- No smoking on the premises, out of consideration for patients trying to quit.

- No alcoholic beverages or recreational drugs on the premises.

- No long or unnecessary personal phone calls.

- Keep voices low at all times, and gently encourage patients or visitors to do the same.

- Maintain a professional, tidy appearance. Wear no perfume, out of consideration for patients who are environmentally sensitive.

- No long personal visits while working.

- Kindly do not offer medical or personal advice to patients without clearing it with me first. I am legally responsible for this.

Note: I generally do not like to talk much in the office, as I talk all day with patients. Please do not take this personally. Also, in the same vein, I usually take lunch alone, away from the office.

Feel free to modify or use this form in your practice.

Protocols

How we follow up with our patients can in itself be therapeutic.

Jennie suffered from panic attacks, anxiety, and insomnia. After an initial intensive course of treatment, we were able to manage her symptoms with treatment once a month, then once every three months. However, we found that if she left my office without having scheduled her next appointment, her symptoms would return within a few days. Simply having the appointment on the books kept her symptoms at bay.

Having a follow-up visit scheduled before the patient leaves the office is often helpful in establishing a feeling of partnership, safety, and stability that is healing, especially for patients who suffer from anxiety or insomnia. Practitioners are often hesitant to clearly tell their patients what they—the practitioner—feels would be best for them, especially when it comes to how frequently the patient should come in for follow-ups. We're concerned it may seem like we are scratching for money. But we need to clearly state when we think a patient should come back for a follow-up. This is not about the money. It is about helping the patient feel secure and offering sufficient support. All too often, if a patient leaves the office without a follow-up appointment scheduled, she feels like she has been cut loose, is on her own, is not entirely clear what she is supposed to do, and is overwhelmed. Her nervous system does not get the support and rest it may so desperately need. While not being aggressive, the practitioner needs to be clear. I would make it a policy not to let a new patient leave the office without making a follow-up appointment, unless it is clear that they do not need or want one, or they have logistical reasons for waiting to schedule one. This follow-up could be scheduled for six months out, but just knowing it is on the books can serve as part of the treatment.

If our environment, the people who work there with us, and how we conduct our business all support the healing process, the jobs of both the doctor and patient are easier.

13 Working with or after Other Practitioners

When a patient consults with a practitioner after seeing many others *and* declares that they were all incompetent, dangerous, or outright quacks, but *you* are different, *you* are what he has been looking for, the odds are that you will join the ranks of those maligned souls sooner or later.

There are several good reasons a patient may have seen many different practitioners. That fact alone is not enough to raise a red flag. It is the declaration of the other practitioners' incompetence, negligence, or quackery that is cause for concern. Probably all practitioners make mistakes. Some more serious than others. If we are in practice long enough, especially if it is a busy practice, we are bound to make some. Even lots of them. It is possible our new patient has been unlucky enough to have seen a string of practitioners who have made grievous errors, but it is unlikely that the entire parade that preceded you was incompetent or worse.

It is my goal and practice to avoid criticizing other practitioners and their advice, even if I disagree with it, and especially if a patient is seeing them or seeking their counsel concurrently with mine. If I agree to have an ongoing therapeutic relationship with a patient who has nothing good to say about previous practitioners, I do so carefully.

Sometimes it can be very beneficial for a patient to see multiple practitioners at the same time, especially if each practitioner is focusing on a different aspect of the patient's health. For example, if a patient is seeing a chiropractor for pain, a massage therapist for muscle tension, and an Ayurvedic practitioner for lifestyle and diet counseling, that could be an easy team to integrate. If, however, a patient gets conflicting advice from different practitioners on the same aspect of his health, it is hard for him to know what to implement or whom to trust. If there is something I think the patient is doing that will truly sabotage her moving in a healthy direction, I may suggest she work exclusively with her other practitioners, and if she chooses, she can always come see me afterward. Otherwise, as long as there are no significant differences or threats to a healthy direction, I will work with the patient to form a treatment strategy together.

14 Turning Away Patients

There is a Sanskrit word, *gati*, which means the same as the English word "gait." In the same way that different animals or human beings have their own particular gait, each relationship has its own nature, or *gati*. This can change over time, but if we are paying attention, we may be able to feel whether the *gati* of our relationship with a potential patient feels conducive to a productive, effective, and harmonious outcome or not.

In some medical professions and jurisdictions, it is legally difficult to discharge a patient, so it is worth careful consideration about whether we are well matched for a positive therapeutic relationship before we commit to it.

Because my guru once told me that a physician should always think she can find the cure for the pain of the patient, I used to think that even if I doubted that a potential patient and I were a good match, it was my duty to treat whoever came to me.

That changed with Paul. At our initial consultation, a couple of things happened. First, I realized that Paul was likely addicted to alcohol and marijuana. He admitted to using both, and told me straightaway that he had no intention of changing those habits in any way. Then, after listing the deficiencies of all the practitioners that he'd seen before, Paul declared that he and I would "get along just fine." He held my hand a little too long when we shook hands goodbye. I had a strong feeling that it was likely that another practitioner—one with more training in treating addictions—would be a better fit for this patient. But since it was my belief that I should treat anybody who came to me, I tried to sort out my discomfort on my own, went against my strong instinct, and accepted Paul as a patient.

For the first few months, the relationship went well enough. But eventually Paul began to call my work number more often, and when he couldn't get me, he found my home phone number and began to call at inappropriate hours and without proper cause. He ignored the boundaries I was setting. I changed my phone number. He began to make veiled threats. I had to discharge him from my practice very carefully. In the end, legal action was required to bring resolution to a situation that had become enormously stressful.

It cost me so much in legal counsel and fees and—above all—stress, I became afraid of my patients for a while. I considered closing my practice and occasionally considered, more than fleetingly, trading it for a job that—in my perception, at least—carried less weighty responsibility: a job like a cashier at a local health food store or a house cleaner. I thought of guru Ravidas, who was a cobbler, and Kabir, a weaver, and my own guru, a farmer. And I deeply appreciated the necessity, integrity, and beauty of those professions.

It took a few years for the situation with Paul to resolve, and for me to regain trust in the rightness of the work I had pursued and trained for in my life. It took reading inspirational works written by saints and students of love and life every night and sometimes multiple times a day to support and regain a healthy perspective on life and indeed, my own health. It took the support and patience of my husband and friends. It took everything I knew, and still it exacted a significant toll before it was resolved.

Had I listened to my instinct that I was not the right practitioner for Paul, I would have referred him right away to a male practitioner with more training in treating addiction. After that experience, I revised my understanding of my guru's words. Just because we may think we *can* help someone, this does not mean it is our responsibility to do so. In reality, it may be *more* helpful for the patient (and the practitioner) if we do not accept those with whom we feel uncomfortable, or who need a practitioner with specialized training in their condition.

Based on my new understanding, I developed a protocol. When a patient made an initial appointment, they were told that during their first visit, we would consider if we were the right fit. In a sense, we were interviewing each other for the job. If we were a good match, we would agree to work together for a while and then re-evaluate. If not, I would suggest where or who else might provide them better or more appropriate care. Using this protocol, I did not turn away lots of people. It was rare for me to turn anybody away, in fact. But it did give me a strategy that was better for both of us if I did decide to turn someone away.

When I accepted someone as a patient, I might spend as much as an hour a month with them. I might know them for years, be in their lives through births, deaths, marriages, divorces, graduations, career changes, etc. Honestly, I have friends I don't get to see as much.

So, when considering if a potential patient and I have the right *gati* for a good therapeutic relationship, I would consider whether this was a person I would like to spend six to 12 hours a year with. Is this someone I would like to know for years to come? If the answer was, "no," I would consider who might be a better fit as a practitioner. I had a file of names of specialists—ones who worked with addiction, or who might be more adept or trained in areas of treatment I was less equipped to address. If I felt that I was not a good fit as a practitioner for a patient, I would say something like, "While I appreciate the time you took to fill out your intake form and meet with me, I feel that another practitioner would be more beneficial for you. I have a list of names."

This did not mean that I referred out every patient who struggled with addiction. Some practitioners talk about having a policy that if their patients don't do what they tell them—like quit drinking or quit eating sugar—they refuse to continue working with them. Though I contemplated such a policy, I did not adopt it. When it came down to it, if it was right to be in a therapeutic relationship with a patient, it felt right to have patience. If I was tempted to become frustrated with the pace at which they were changing or healing, I would remember how many times my guru told me to do something and I still didn't do it—yet he never gave up on me.

When I had a patient who simply couldn't or wasn't ready to give up a detrimental habit, I would treat them and then every six months or so have a conversation about the issue. I would say something like, "So, I want to make sure we are not just wasting time. We both know you are still _____-ing, and that is still taking a toll on your health, and we know that nothing we do here together can reverse that. I don't want to waste your money or time. Do you feel you are still getting benefit from this relationship?" If the answer was yes, and it always was, we kept going. This served the purpose of taking stock, reminding each other that we knew that there was an important issue still on the table, and offering compassion and empathy.

On the other hand, it is worth keeping in mind these words that Edward Kentish, L.Ac. shared: "Don't work harder than your patient." It is not necessarily our failing if patients don't quit a bad habit or change course in their lives. We can only do our best to support the changes, cultivate good habits in our own lives, and accept the outcome.

15 Tell the Truth

Jack belonged to the martini-lunch generation. Over the course of the day and evening, that martini was joined by more drinks. This happened every day and every evening. Jack loved that his doctor would give him a clean bill of health every time he had a check-up—it seems his doctor never checked Jack's blood alcohol level. And since Jack's diabetes was managed, Jack (and, apparently, his doctor) felt he was on solid ground with his health, and did not address the issue of how much he drank.

Andrea lived a few blocks from the tastiest fried food in town, and she ate it daily. She was 60 pounds overweight but got what she described as "a clean bill of health" each time she went for a check-up. When she developed hypertension and gallstones, she was able to control the blood pressure with medication and she had her gall bladder removed. She continued to receive those clean bills of health since all her lab results fell within normal ranges, as long as she took her medication.

In CAM, we generally recognize that good health is more than controlled numbers on lab tests. We generally understand that being overweight or underweight, or suffering from anxiety, digestive discomfort, or addiction to alcohol, cigarettes, sugar, too much fried or processed food, or other harmful substances, are all indicative of a trajectory that is unlikely to land somewhere good. This has nothing to do with moral judgment. For example, it is not that drinking alcohol is "evil." It is that, over time and in excess, it affects the health of the liver and the emotions, increases the risk of many cancers, perpetuates insomnia, and delivers other unhealthy side effects.

If someone comes to us with poor life habits, it may be easier to avoid addressing them in the short term. But that is not serving the long-term health of the patient. It may be more often the case in Western medicine than in CAM that patients seek doctors who will overlook their poor health habits. Ideally, patients are not choosing practitioners who simply tell them what they want to hear, and avoiding ones who will speak the truth. In any case, it is up to us to decide whether this is part of our practice or not. If we want to tell the truth, it can be very effective. Sometimes a direct approach works wonderfully. With other patients, a more subtle approach may work better.

Dr. Joel was a retired surgeon. He was a frequent patient at the Acupuncture student clinic where I worked as a supervisor. The first time I oversaw his treatment, his chart showed that he had been treated for over a year for the same conditions. This is not unheard of, or even uncommon, but is always worth investigating to make sure something is not being missed. The student practitioner working with Dr. Joel told me she had seen him many times, and that he had been smoking large amounts of marijuana as long as he'd been coming in. The stubborn conditions I had noticed were both directly related to this use. The student said she had not been comfortable talking with Dr. Joel about his habit and its consequences.

We went in to see him together, and I explained the situation. I told him, "Dr. Joel, if you choose to continue to smoke this much, I think it unlikely that either of these conditions will go away. I'm not saying you have to quit. I am saying that I think your chances of being cured increase dramatically if you do. If you do not, I am happy to continue supervising treatments, but I think it is important for you to know that these treatments are, at best, simply managing the results of your habit."

About a week later, I passed Dr. Joel in the hallway. He came up to me, gave me a big hug, and thanked me for speaking with him so directly about his habit. He had felt heard, understood, and even respected because of the directness of our interaction.

At about that same time, Jeanne came to see me. During her first consultation, she told me in a very forthright way that she drank a minimum of one bottle of wine each night, and her husband did too, and they loved it. She also told me that she wanted to get pregnant and did not want me to tell her she should quit drinking before conceiving. She said she did not believe the studies, and the doctors who said that drinking would damage her baby.

While there are certainly problems with studies, as we have seen, the studies on this issue are indisputable. Drinking alcohol while pregnant harms the fetus, and thus harms the baby and the person he becomes. But I couldn't tell this to Jeanne. She had already informed me that she was deaf to that line of reasoning.

So we finished the intake and I looked at her tongue and felt her pulses. Not surprisingly, the heavy use of alcohol was affecting her health in specific ways. Toward the end of the consultation I said:

> Jeanne, I respect that you don't want me to tell you to quit drinking for your baby. And I won't. But I will tell you I think you should quit drinking for your own sake. It is clearly beginning to affect your organs and overall health. You have to quit. It is not a question of whether this is going to hurt you or not. It already has. It is just a question of how much. At this point in your life, you could come back from this. I don't see any reason why your organs and tissues cannot regain full health, if you quit. You have to quit.

This was both a direct and indirect approach. It was an indirect way to support her baby, and a direct appeal to her own mortality and instinct for self-preservation. It was not a moral judgment. It was connecting the dots of cause and effect.

Jeanne quit drinking that week. She got pregnant that year, and she and her baby were alcohol-free. As I recall, even her husband reduced or quit his drinking as well. I am aware that this is a surprising story. It is easy to think, in fact, that it would be impossible for someone to change so thoroughly and so quickly. It isn't. Jeanne did it. We will look more at the benefit of brief interventions like this in Chapter 21.

I have often found it tempting to sidestep the truth when dealing with teenagers or young adults. I think we often don't tell them the truth out of fear that we will alienate them. But I think we underestimate the good that can come from telling the truth without judgment or condemnation.

I smoked rather heavily for a couple years when I was a teenager, starting at about age 15. For a couple of years, not a single grown-up confronted me about this. Then one day, my stepmother—a woman I admired and trusted—said something like, "You are such a smart girl. The only thing you do that doesn't fit is the smoking." It wasn't heavy. It was just her observation. I quit shortly after that. Some 30 years later, I still remember the impact those words had on my spirit and my behavior.

There are least three young people with whom I have been very direct about their smoking, once we established a rapport. They were all students of healthcare, in my classes. In each case, they confided in me that they smoked. I confided in them that I smoked, too, as a teenager, and even many years after I quit, I would indulge in the occasional cigarette. Eventually I stopped doing even that, knowing I was tempting fate, given my history, parentage, proclivities and the hazards of smoking. I was very clear with these students about my past, and told them directly, "You have to quit. You just have to quit. It is not a question of whether this is going to hurt you. It is only a question of when and how badly." Then, as I recall, in each case, I broke all the unwritten rules of co-dependent behavior. (In fact, they probably are written down somewhere…) I said with a little humor but also truth, "If you can't do it for you, do it for me."

In each case, I cared very much for the student. And I felt conviction.

In each case, the student quit smoking.

This goes back to the question of communication.

My sister has a friend who says something like this: "If I think I need to say something to someone that might either be difficult for me to say or for them to hear, I pray to God to give me the person, the words, and the opportunity, and I will cooperate." This has helped me on probably hundreds of occasions, both in and outside my practice.

Saying something at the wrong time, or in the wrong way, can act as a poison. Saying the same thing at the right moment in the right way can be wonderful medicine. Being able to tell the difference between the right and wrong time and way takes practice.

At any given moment, it is either right to say something or wrong, or unclear whether it is right or wrong. If it is unclear, I generally go by the rule, "When in doubt, do nothing." Eventually it becomes clear if it is good to say something or not, and then the only question that remains is, do I have the courage to say it or to keep quiet?

I also generally go by my own rule. When I feel emotionally charged about something, try to wait to say anything about it until I no longer do. Take a walk. Drink a tall glass of water. Wait until the charge passes. Then do not be afraid to tell the truth if it becomes clear that it is the right path.

In any case, if we are as centered as we can be, and feel clear, and wait for the right opportunity, telling the truth can be a powerful catalyst for transformation.

16 The Role of Story in Diagnosis, Treatment, and Compliance

The job of the healer is to hear the story and
help the person reweave the story.
DR. ROBERT E. SVOBODA

I have had many students ask some version or another of this question: how do we make patients more compliant?

We don't. Psychology 101 does not go out the window when we start practicing medicine. We don't *make* people feel something, do something, or say something, anymore than they *make* us feel, do, or say anything. Trying to force an outcome or *make* somebody do something violates their freedom.

Thankfully, there is a difference between trying to make a patient do something and sharing what inspires us, telling them what has worked for us or others, and working together toward finding a healthier direction for them. Even if this is just a baby step in that direction.

Jesse had a number of health issues and poor habits. When, at the urging of his wife, he went to see prominent Ayurvedic physician Dr. Robert Svoboda, he was dubious that he would receive any benefit because he was unwilling to change his habits. He showed up and had the consultation. Later, Jesse described to me how the session ended. "It came to the part when Dr. Svoboda was going to tell me what to do. He asked me, 'Are you willing to give up X?' I said, 'Probably not.' He said, 'Would you take any herbs?' I said, 'Probably not.' He said, 'Would you change your diet?' I said, 'Probably not.' Then he asked, 'Would you be willing to give up coffee?' And I said, 'I could probably do that.' I was impressed by his flexibility and his non-judgmental approach to finding *something* I could do. So I made that one change, and it did make a difference in my health."

I use the terms "compliance" and "non-compliance" in this book because they are common terms in the medical profession, and we all know what they mean. But aren't they just a bit patronizing? Don't they clearly imply that we know what is best for a patient? Yet, as we have seen, there is very little we do know.

When a patient comes to us, we take his health history. Let's look at that word, "history." If we break it down, it is, "his story." We listen to his story. We combine his story with what we perceive from his living story—what we hear, see, smell, and feel from him and with him. We consider this constellation of seemingly disparate pieces of data in light of everything we have studied, read, learned, and experienced before. Looking at the constellation, we create our own story with its own meaning. We call this story a "diagnosis" and it informs and directs another story: our treatment strategy, prescriptions, and pronounced prognosis, no matter what modality of medicine we practice. An elegant story is one that reflects careful listening, and redirects the patient's story, if necessary.

I don't mean "story" in a negative sense, like we are lying. I mean it in a positive sense, whereby we work to find meaning and to visualize the path that led the patient to trouble and the path that may lead them to health. A patient's alignment with the perceptions—we could say the "stories" of the physician—is strongly associated with positive recovery.[1] When both doctor and patient agree on a story—a diagnosis and treatment plan—we have a collaborative rather than a hierarchical relationship. We have a sense of shared perceptions and decisions. We may adopt parts of the story that aid hope, health and recovery, and starve the parts that perpetuate ill health of one sort or another. We have a partnership. Together we can "see" the way out, the way towards less pain, more health. Most likely, the patient feels a sense of empowerment.

This feeling of collaboration can increase the sense of control a patient has over his own life and health and sometimes death. Studies have shown positive correlations between this sense of control and recovery from illness, tolerance of pain, improved daily functioning, better mental health, decreased hospital stays, and even decreased tumor growth.[2]

Once both patient and physician are in agreement and alignment with the diagnosis, treatment strategy, and recommended lifestyle and dietary changes, the patient often has a strong need for support to stay the new course. Different personalities may respond better to different types of support. A nervous or anxious patient may be best supported through comforting and encouraging words. An inquisitive, intellectual patient may best be supported through education and inspiration. A lethargic patient may best be supported the way a sports coach or drill sergeant would motivate her team or new recruits.

Sometimes people have better outcomes when they seek out the company of someone else, or a group of people who are trying to do the same thing they are. This could take the form of attending Alcoholics Anonymous meetings, spiritual or religious gatherings, group or individual personal therapy, yoga classes, the gym, or other supportive communities. Deeply considering how much support a patient is likely to require, what type of support will best match their nature, and how to facilitate this support can have a strong bearing on the outcome.

Our own confidence in a treatment plan can be infectious. For example, castor oil packs can be incredibly good medicine for many disorders, but they need to be left on for about 90 minutes. When practitioners or students learn this, they sometimes exclaim that there is no way patients will comply with this treatment. Yet I have had probably hundreds, possibly thousands, of patients who *have* complied—and reaped the benefits. It seems to me there are several reasons for compliance in the face of this sizeable commitment of time. One is that pain is a serious motivator, so patients are willing to take time if it means the pain will go away. Another is the strong confidence of the practitioner in the story: the diagnosis and treatment plan. Perceiving this, the patient is convinced to try it, she sees the results, and gains even more confidence to proceed in a healthy direction.

There is a concept, "narrative medicine," that explores the importance of patients' stories, as well as employing storytelling in the art of medicine. It is an idea whose time seems to have come. Again. In June 2007, Dr. Lewis Mehl-Madrona's wonderful book, *Narrative Medicine: The Use of History and Story in the Healing Process,* was published. About seven-and-a-half months later, *Narrative Medicine: Honoring the Stories of Illness,* by Dr. Rita Charon, founder and Executive Director of the Program in Narrative Medicine at Columbia University, was published.

Dr. Mehl-Madrona rekindles the ancient knowledge and reverence for stories, and helps us understand how to work with them more consciously. They can also help us tell truth in creative ways, as we can sometimes hear stories of others' trials, victories, struggles, and resolutions more easily than being told something in a direct way. Stories have long been part of healing in traditional culture and, while we may think of the traditional healer employing storytelling in the healing process, patients' stories are equally important. Dr. Charon's program brings stories into the classrooms of medical students, where they carefully read literature and write reflective works, to hone their ability to listen to patients' stories more carefully and effectively. While Dr. Mehl-Madrona and Dr. Charon have somewhat different approaches, they both explore the role of listening to, and telling, stories in medicine and healing.

When the stories and beliefs of the physician and patient are aligned, the patient is more likely to trust the doctor, the treatment, and the treatment modality. When that happens, the chances of a positive outcome improve. If the physician and patient are not in alignment, these chances drop, even if the treatment strategy is otherwise appropriate.[3]

17 Confidence vs. Cockiness

Attention is often given to the role that a patient's belief in a particular treatment plays in its efficacy. But there is an equally fascinating question regarding the role that the physician's belief plays in the outcome. It has been demonstrated that the physician's belief in a particular therapy can and does affect the outcome for a patient, *even in double-blind studies.*[1]

For example, researcher Jerry Solfvin closely examined how the beliefs of doctors affected three double-blind studies conducted on the use of Vitamin E in treating pain associated with coronary artery disease. One doctor leading one of the studies enthusiastically believed in the power of Vitamin E to benefit the patients, while the two doctors leading the other studies did not. The results of these double-blind studies matched the doctors' beliefs. The enthusiastic doctor found Vitamin E significantly more effective than the placebo,[2] whereas the other two doctors found no effect from Vitamin E.[3]

Here's another example Solfvin writes about. In the 1950s there were conflicting reports about an early tranquilizing drug called meprobamate. A double-blind study was designed whereby one administering physician felt positive and enthusiastic about the drug, and another was skeptical about its value. Neither the administering physicians nor the patients knew whether the patients were receiving placebos or meprobamate. Nor were they even aware that they were involved in the experiment. The results were that the drug proved more effective for the patients of the enthusiastic doctor but no better than the placebo for the patients of the skeptical doctor.[4] This study was repeated three times in different locations, and replicated in two out of the three. After his research, Solfvin concluded that double-blind test results are influenced by the administering physicians' beliefs.[5]

If our belief has the power to enhance or diminish the chances of a positive outcome for a patient, then what we believe is mightily important. If true, we should only prescribe therapies or courses of action we believe in, or at least have hope in. My guru told me that a doctor should always believe she can find the goodness, the cure, for the patient's pain. Believing this conveys and instills confidence in the patient and, it seems, shapes the outcome.

Knowing how little we actually know, how can we be confident? I once knew a man, a fellow disciple of my guru, and a reportedly brilliant surgeon. At his eulogy, his son shared that his father had a specific ritual he would perform at the beginning of every surgical shift. He would look at his hands and say, "Okay, Master, what are you going to do with these hands today?" The surgeon believed that his master was working through his hands, so he had confidence in the work he was about to do. His confidence was not in his own knowledge, which, being human, was limited. His confidence was in his master. His patients didn't have to know that. Their experience simply was that their surgeon was confident.

For reasons too lengthy to relay here, my sister Sam and I were standing outside the doors of Indira Gandhi International Airport in Delhi, India, about to catch a flight back to New York, where Sam lived. Sam was seven-and-a-half months pregnant. And she had just gone into labor. Not Braxton Hicks contractions. Labor.

Now, had I not previously spent time as a patient in a hospital in Delhi, and had I no idea of what is involved to keep a premature baby alive and safe, maybe I would have felt more relaxed about this situation. Maybe not. In any case, relaxed would describe neither Sam's state nor mine.

After considering briefly whether to hail a cab to the hospital or continue through customs, it was clear to us that we would rather see this baby born in France, on our layover there (and closer to New York) than in the hospital in Delhi (no disrespect meant to the fine physicians and facilities available there). Having lived in India, being able to speak some Hindi, and having some understanding of medicine—also not being in labor myself—Sam was looking to me for direction.

I sensed that the only way to truly calm her was to feel calm myself. I did not feel calm. I felt about as *not* calm as I had ever felt in my life. As I placed our luggage on the X-ray conveyer belt (the first of many steps one must take in the Indira Gandhi airport), I prayed to my guru. I must say here that although my guru maintained that perfect saints do not perform miracles, it had been my experience on occasion that they do. That is, if completely changing a deeply held perspective or state of being can be called a miracle. To me, it seems miraculous. My—well, *our*—miracle that day was that by the time our luggage emerged on the other side of the X-ray belt, I was calm and sure. Seeing an elephant transformed into a squirrel would not have impressed me as more miraculous.

Right there, in the middle of the bustling, chaotic, loud airport hall, Sam and I looked at each other. I asked her to do some exercises with me. We did a few minutes of breathing and visualization exercises, and her labor stopped. It stopped. She continued to quietly and continuously do the exercises while I navigated us through the many final steps before getting on the plane.

Her beautiful boy was born a couple of months later. In New York.

That day in the airport, Sam and I both felt the power of confidence (also the power of breathing exercises, but that is a story for a different day). We can always find something honest to be confident about.

We can consciously cultivate confidence. Perhaps not in our own limited—sometimes meager—abilities, but in Something Bigger Than Ourselves. This is one of the most important aspects of medicine I know.

In less lofty but very real ways, we can build confidence in the next step we will take. We can build confidence that things will become clear. We can build confidence through inspiration gleaned from our studies, textbooks, scriptures, professors, lectures, our personal experience, and our intuition as our senses are refined.

There is a caution here, though. While confidence may support good health and results, becoming cocky can be dangerous.

I have had my share of professors and teachers who had reputations for arrogance or cockiness. It is possible that their expertise was sometimes confused with arrogance, but it is also possible that they were indeed arrogant or cocky. In any case, I have personally learned to overlook the distasteful aspects of those qualities, because often these teachers were arrogant for a reason: they had great experience and got great results. They knew plenty—which means they knew some things that would be valuable for me to learn. I have found it very useful to pay close attention when there is perceived or reputed arrogance.

While the consequences of cockiness may be less obvious or severe with a professor, it is dangerous in medical practice. I may have made more mistakes in my practice due to momentary cockiness than anything else. It is easy to succumb to this when a patient comes in complaining of a symptom or disorder that we have treated successfully many times. It is easy at this moment to think something along the lines of, *Ah ha! I know this. This is easy. This is XYZ. One acupuncture treatment and a couple weeks of ABC and she will be good to go.* When we've had 99 great outcomes, of course the 100th will be great too, right? Not necessarily. Whether this is Murphy's Law, the dark sense of humor of the Powers That Be, or a fallacy, it certainly seemed to me that the times I got cocky, I would inevitably discover that it was a dangerous trap to fall into.

Getting cocky about the 100th patient leads us to look less carefully, be less present, miss something important, prescribe more quickly, or offer somewhat cavalier treatment. I can't remember all the times I did this, and I am grateful the consequences were usually not too severe. They were just bad enough to wake me up to the possibility that they could have been much worse.

Cockiness suggests arrogance, and patients report less satisfaction and poorer results with doctors they perceive as arrogant. They also sue them more frequently than doctors they perceive to be empathetic.[1] A good thing to remember.

Because, as we established in Part I, we don't really *know* very much, it is a good idea to proceed with caution with every patient, even when we've seen a symptom or a treatment work "a million times," lest we err on the side of cockiness and invite trouble.

The main way to avoid cockiness is to cultivate humility (which we talked about in Part I) and remember our own vast limitations.

It is also helpful to remember the vulnerability of our patient. My friend and colleague, Pamela Kentish, L.Ac., recently reminded me how humbling and beautiful it is that patients ask for help and place their trust in us, and what a responsibility that is. It is probably impossible to feel the honest weight of this responsibility and be cocky at the same time.

If we cultivate a healthy sense of our own limitations, add that to our faith or confidence in Something Larger Than Ourselves, and maintain confidence that we can find a cure for the patient's pain (even if he is dying, we can find something to make him more comfortable), then we may be able to treat with confidence, without indulging cockiness.

18 Great Loss and Suffering

One thing I have found again and again with people who have experienced great loss is that they are often in a heightened state of receptivity to love, deep communication, and sharing their grief. It is often those of us who have not recently, or ever, suffered such a loss that are uncomfortable with it. We can distance ourselves from people by thinking thoughts like, "I can't possibly understand their grief because I haven't experienced it." While this may well be true, it does not mean we cannot offer empathy, love, and deep human connection.

My friend Diane's eight-year-old son, Donald, had cancer and was fighting for his life. Donald was in and out of hospitals for four years before he died. During this time, I was living on the other side of the country, and rarely had the opportunity to see Diane or Donald. But there was a website dedicated to Donald where those of us who loved him could get updates and leave messages.

About three years into the experience, Diane posted a note asking us not to say certain things in our messages. I don't remember her list exactly, but it started with things that seemed pretty clearly unhelpful, like, "Don't tell me Donald is going to a better place. He is not. The best place for him is in his mother's arms." I felt pretty confident I wouldn't say something like that, but as I read on, I remember feeling less confident in my ability to say *anything* that wouldn't hurt, let alone help. There were things like, "Don't tell me I look good," and "Don't tell me I look like shit." I also wondered what I could say to Diane, since I do not have children and so could not begin to understand what it would feel like to lose a child. Maybe it would be better for me to say nothing, I thought. But when I considered it deeply, I saw that this line of thinking was creating a division between us. We were two human beings who cared about each other and were capable of empathy. I decided it was more important for me to be in touch than to withdraw out of fear that I might make things worse. I remember simply sending her love, over and over and over. The subject line of my messages was almost always just "love."

Years have passed since Donald's death, and Diane and I remain dear friends. She has never pushed me away, saying I couldn't possibly understand what she went through. She didn't have to say that. We both know it and we both bridged the distance—we reached past any distance to embrace each other's hearts.

About a year ago, I reminded Diane of that list, and asked her if there was something that *was* good to hear during those days. What would be on her "Do say this" list? She paused, and then said, "'I'm sorry.' 'I'm sorry' was good to hear."

Another dear friend lost her 21-year-old son suddenly and tragically. This friend, too, bridged the gap with me, and we have met in waterfalls of pain and stood there, drenched. One day she volunteered that she just couldn't hear "I'm sorry" anymore, from anyone. It was all she was hearing sometimes. And it hurt. She felt that "I'm sorry" was all about the person saying it. It was something *they* felt and it didn't help her at all.

There is no manual of what to say to someone who has experienced excruciating loss. If there is one that I don't know about, I expect it can't tell us the perfect thing to say anyway. To one person, "I'm sorry" might be one of the only things that makes sense. To someone else, it hurts.

This is one of the reasons it is so important to refine our senses. If we can communicate on a deeper level than words, the exact words may not matter as much. When we don't let suffering divide us, and we commit to hearing, seeing, and feeling more deeply, we can meet there, in that place that words can't reach—that horrible, real, sometimes grace-filled, beautiful, tender, and exquisite reality.

19 Cake or Death? Choosing Hope

"Where there is life, there is hope," is no less true
for being a cliché; faith and hope, the physician's
allies, must be reinforced whenever possible.
DR. ROBERT E. SVOBODA

John had had a massive hemorrhagic stroke. As he lay in critical care on the first day, I stood with his daughter, Rachel, by his side. A physician came in, and Rachel asked what the chances were that her father would survive and be able to walk out of the hospital as the man she knew. The doctor's face showed his struggle. He was unable to say a word. Then he began to cry and left the room, leaving the family with the impression that they must prepare for the worst.

A couple hours later, another physician entered. Rachel asked him the same question. This doctor said he thought John would be able to leave the hospital with some residual right-side weakness.

Both doctors had seen the same scans and tests, and, as if the possible outcomes were listed on a menu, each had chosen one. From that time on, Rachel, her family, and I, understood that we, too, could choose from the menu. What to choose? I am reminded of comedian Eddie Izzard's sketch, "Cake or Death?" Um. Cake, please.

While we truly appreciated the humanity and empathy of the first doctor, who clearly cared about John's fate, we found it a better strategy for us to choose the prediction of the hopeful doctor. We chose cake. Indeed, the prediction of the optimistic doctor was more accurate in the end.

Whether or not the prediction of the optimistic doctor affected John's outcome—and we have seen (in Chapter 17) that it certainly could have—his approach certainly made the waiting period for his family, and for John once he regained consciousness, more bearable. I'm not sure there is a difference between hope and false hope. There may just be hope. And hope is a far better place to live than hopelessness.

A cursory search for the connection between optimism and health reveals multiple studies connecting the two in positive ways. For example, optimism has been found to be a positive factor in recovery for heart patients, whereby optimistic patients experience a faster rate of recovery during their hospitalization and a faster rate of return to normal activities and good quality of life after discharge.[1] In 2011, Researchers at Duke University Medical Center found that optimism was associated not only with better short-term recovery but with overall survival and health over the long term. In their study, they followed more than 2,800 heart patients over 15 years and found that those who were even modestly optimistic about their treatment and recovery were significantly more likely to be alive after 15 years than moderately pessimistic patients with similar conditions.[2] Optimism is neither a practice of denial, nor is it a reflection of naivete. It is choosing to perceive and attend to the positive aspects of a situation.

It is beneficial for patients to find people—including doctors—who carry faith and hope for them.

In Chapter 17, we looked at the role of the doctor's confidence and beliefs, in outcome. Confidence is related closely to hope. It is contagious. If we have hopeful, optimistic outlooks, this can support the same in patients. And then we see better outcomes.

My guru told me a doctor should always think he will be able to find the goodness and the cure of the pain of the person. He didn't say we should think this 90 percent of the time, and then the rest of the time tell our patients that there is nothing we can do. And he did not say the doctor should always believe he can *cure* the patient. He said we should think we can *find* the cure for the pain of the patient. If we are familiar with authoritative texts, have cautiously studied research on the treatments and herbs we use, and haven't found solutions in the usual places, we can look outside the familiar. We can have faith that there is something that can cure the pain, and we trust in our sincerity in trying to find it.

I understand that in the New Testament of the Bible, the word usually translated as "sin"—that most weighty and doom-saying word many of us have come to find distasteful—is a translation of a Greek word *hamartia,* an archery term that simply means "missing the mark." So sinning is simply not hitting the bull's eye. I have come to see that, if my bull's eye is a positive outlook and I focus on anything but that, I am missing the mark. I am literally sinning, according to that definition of sin.

This is not to say that people always get better and never die. It is to say that there is always something positive to focus on.

Phil was dying of cancer. When it was clear that his death was near, a dear friend planned to visit him and was to arrive on Monday. Phil passed away on Sunday, missing his friend by a day. From one point of view this was a tragedy—something Phil was dearly looking forward to that did not come to pass. From another point of view, his friend gave him something hopeful to focus on at a time where hope was a scarce commodity. Phil spent his last days looking forward to something instead of fighting against something else. He passed away in peace.

Hope is good. What is not helpful is this: empty promises or declarations about a future we can't predict, unless we are fully prepared to stand by such a promise. When we are in the throes of suffering or fear, having someone say, *don't worry, dear. Everything is going to be okay,* can feel incredibly alienating. How can that person possibly know everything is going to be okay? We can't honestly say, "Debra, you can beat this cancer." Even feeling attached to that, or some outcome, distorts our ability to be fully present to perceive what is happening and the reality of the person in front of us.

Robert had been through intensive chemotherapy for cancer. The chemotherapy had not been successful in treating the cancer, and had weakened his heart. When he was hospitalized for congestive heart failure, and his heart recovered, Robert's cardiologist was optimistic and cheerful. He did not think Robert needed home healthcare or hospice care. From his point of view, Robert had suffered some heart issues, which were now better. He didn't spend more than five minutes with Robert in a single visit. He didn't see that the cancer had ravaged and weakened him. He looked at the tests that measured the condition of Robert's heart and, since those were within normal range, he was satisfied. He left the room, with Robert's family feeling unseen and unheard, but mostly upset that Robert had not really been seen or heard. When Robert passed away about a week later, the cardiologist was the only person who was surprised.

Thrusting hope at someone like it's a lollipop may demonstrate ignorance of how the person is feeling or of what their condition really is.

Even if the ultimate outcome is death, we can take the time to perceive the patient and reality as fully as possible and as well as we can and, together, wait patiently to discover the hope that is real. When we don't go frantically searching for hope, and we simply wait for it, something real and tangible may arrive to represent hope.

For example, even in extreme circumstances, there is a very real possibility that we can make someone more comfortable, take the time to learn what their goals are, and help them achieve those goals. The goals of the elderly, for example, may shift away from attachment to curing medical conditions and more towards avoiding falls and enhancing quality of life. We can also sometimes offer patients physical, emotional, or mental comfort—even if momentarily—when they are with us. Doing this can serve as a reminder, even a small one, of what health or hope feels like. This gives a patient a glimpse into what is possible, and what they can shoot for. Experiencing even momentary relief can help a patient find hope and peace.

When survival or prognosis statistics for a given disease do not appear to be on the side of hope, we need to apply at least as much cautionary skepticism to those results as to our patient's condition. Prognostic and survival statistics, even if they do not suffer from the plague of factors that may skew study results, have their limitations. These sorts of statistics tell us something about the severity of the disease or condition a person suffers from, but nothing about the person who suffers from it. Two individuals may have the same condition, say, a broken hip. But if one patient is a young, healthy individual and the other is 95, the prognosis is likely to be very different indeed. The same would be the case if one patient is optimistic and the other pessimistic, as we have seen.

Consider this study, which looked at the relapse rate for women with metastatic breast cancer. We could read the stated results that

80 percent of women suffering with this disease die of it, and be tempted to convey a sense of hopelessness to our patients. Or we could see—in the same study—that "the longest interval to relapse has been 23.5 years, and 18 percent of those who relapsed did so more than 10 years later."[3]

As physicians, we are often told that we have to be realistic. But considering that we truly do not know what outcome our patient is going to have, we have a choice about where we put our focus. There is a menu. We can choose cake.

Introduction to Chapters 20–24

The following chapters on sexual abuse, addictions, mental illness, eating disorders, and domestic violence have a few things in common. Each of these conditions may require a referral to, or at least concurrent treatment with, a professional trained in the issue in order for the patient to move forward in a healthy direction. Indeed, such a referral may be required to save the patient's life.

Each of these disorders can be present in anyone from any social or financial class, any race, status, or caste. Patients may also suffer from more than one of these conditions concurrently. A patient suffering from any one of these disorders could walk into our practice any day. It is easy to think that because it hasn't happened yet, it never will. If you have a busy practice, one day it is likely to. One day, a patient with a potentially fatal addiction will come to you. Or someone suffering from an eating disorder or domestic abuse. Or someone so depressed they are contemplating suicide. Or someone who was sexually assaulted, last week, last year, or 30 years ago.

Whether or not we have lost loved ones to any of these conditions, we may remember how surprised or upset we were hearing about the ultimate toll they exacted on others, like those brilliant actors and souls Philip Seymour Hoffman and Robin Williams. It is better to be prepared than surprised. We can't all be trained in how to treat every one of these disorders, but if we learn something about them, have a few tools to use, and a list of resources to hand to these patients, we may be able to help them find the comfort and treatment they need. And this could save a life.

It is not my intention to teach anyone how to treat these conditions, but rather to explore ways we can think about them and bring their seriousness to our awareness so we are more likely to recognize them and either receive training ourselves or refer patients to other appropriate, trained therapists.

20 Sexual Abuse

This is a big topic. There are specialists who receive training in understanding, support, and counseling around sexual abuse. This is not training that every practitioner receives. Nor is it within the scope of this book to offer specialized education in this area, but there are a couple things that may be helpful for all of us to be aware of, considering the prevalence of sexual abuse. In the US alone, someone is the victim of attempted or committed rape every 107 seconds.[1] In their lifetime, one in every six American women, and one in every 33 men, has been such a victim.[2] If you are in a busy medical practice, you likely have many patients with such a history. It is a pity if we are ignorant of this, or of what behavior may help or aggravate these cases.

As we looked at briefly in Chapter 3 on inference, it is rather an open secret among practitioners who work with many women patients that the longer the history of gynecological or urogenital tract afflictions, the more likely it is that the woman has a history of sexual abuse. I have not seen any studies about this, but I have seen it myself many times, and had it reinforced by the reports of so many practitioners, that it is an observation that carries weight with me. I don't automatically assume a history of abuse if there is a history of gynecological complications, but I consider it a real possibility.

When I was first in practice, I would look for confirmation of this association. I felt the consultation time and space was a safe place for such an experience to be expressed or confirmed, and I felt there might be benefit to doing so. One day, when I was supervising a student clinic, the student was consulting with her patient, a woman with a long history of gynecological disorders. In what I thought was a delicate manner, I enquired of the woman if she remembered any history of abuse. She said she had no such history. Later I found out she was disturbed I had asked her.

Most physicians want to have a positive effect on their patients, and it can feel shocking to do otherwise. These experiences can lead us to some soul searching. I thought about this woman's feedback for a long time, and came to a conclusion that has guided my practice since. It is not necessary to either ask or receive verbal confirmation of a history of physical or sexual abuse. Such a revelation neither needs to be solicited nor discouraged. If it happens on its own, that is fine—and possibly therapeutic—but it is not always necessary for healing and, if solicited, may feel or actually be injurious.

It might be blasphemous to say this, as a practitioner of "holistic" medicine claiming to treat individuals in unique ways, but the course of treatment may be the same whether a patient discloses a history of abuse or not. We address any maladies while conveying sensitivity and respect for the patient through any communication or physical contact. For example, we could treat a broken arm without knowing its cause. Whether the arm was broken out of violence or because of an accident, we still approach the arm and the person with love, respect, and awareness of their whole being. While it might be healing for the patient to express the cause, we ourselves may not need to hear it vocalized.

I think a stance of, "Don't ask, but be receptive if someone volunteers sensitive information," is applicable to other clinical but sensitive issues like libido or sexual practices, as well. No need to ask unless there is a strong need to know.

This isn't necessarily a hard and fast rule, however. The woman who was offended by my question was not a patient of mine. We didn't have a history together. It is possible that there might come a time with a patient when it would be okay to ask this question. But in my experience, it is good to have it become very clear that this is an important question to ask.

There are other questions not to ask.

A hurtful question in the case of sexual assault or abuse would be some version of this: "What did you do to invite this?" It might take the form of one of these: "What were you wearing?" "How late were you out?" "Where were you?" "Were you drinking?" "Were you being flirtatious?" Anything that implies or suggests complicity or places responsibility on the woman or man assaulted, instead of the person who violated them, can place more burden on an already burdened spirit. It could be the case that a young woman made a poor choice to get drunk and walk in a bad part of town, but that still doesn't mean it is her fault that she was assaulted or abused.

When we encounter things outside our own experience, it may be easy to ask questions borne of ignorance. At best, our patients will have the presence of mind to tolerate our ignorance and the patience to educate us. At worst, doing so will confirm our ignorance, alienate the patient, and possibly add more damage, hurt, and loneliness to someone already too familiar with them.

Along with ignorant questions, there are ignorant things we can say. It might seem like it should go without saying that sexual innuendo does not belong in a doctor's office, but unfortunately, it may actually need to be said. While there can be a beautiful, comfortable, and trusting emotional intimacy between doctor and patient, it is not an invitation for sexual innuendo.

Leslie considered herself a woman comfortable with her sexuality and she enjoyed flirting. She told me this story. She was seeing a (male) physical therapist for exercises after knee surgery. He asked her to remove her pants and get into a gown, in order to do the exercises. She jokingly said, "Now we're really going to have fun!" She shared with me that, even though she meant this to be full of sexual innuendo, she was still taken aback when the therapist went along with it and responded, "Well this day is about to get a whole lot better!" She suddenly felt shocked, sad, and less trusting. She felt a distance open up between her and the therapist that replaced the trust and appropriate intimacy she had felt before this brief exchange.

Even if patients are comfortable with their relationship to and with sexuality, and even if they joke in a sexual way, it can be damaging for the practitioner to be an accomplice in this. Even if sexual innuendo or flirtation seems to work for a doctor outside the office, it does not foster safe or appropriate intimacy *in* the office, *even if it seems like patients are okay with it.* It is possible that some are. Many are not and will not want to say so. If we bring sexual language or innuendo into this relationship, the best that can happen is that we are indulged or forgiven. The worst can range from alienating patients, to offending them, to damaging them if they have experienced sexual abuse in the past, and it is likely to sabotage appropriate intimacy, even if the doctor is not aware of it.

What Can We Do?

We can leave sexual innuendo out of our relationships with our patients, and if a woman or man discloses a history of sexual abuse, we can consider responses like the following:

- Treat them with great sensitivity and respect, as we would any patient.

- After the disclosure, pause. Allow some space and some quiet until she is ready to continue. It is not necessary to hug away the pain or to try to fix it, though saying something in empathetic acknowledgement can be helpful. A friend who founded and ran a newsletter for women who were abused in childhood told me it is helpful to say something simple like, "I am so sorry this happened to you." I found this to be true in my experience as well. Being present, non-judgmental, calm, and committing to seeing, hearing, and feeling deeply can ease the experience of being alone in pain, and can replace shame with relief.

- Provide a list of practitioners who specialize in treatment or counseling in this area, if we don't have that training ourselves.

- Provide resources, such as these listed below.

Resources

- *Rape and sexual assault crisis centers.* Look up your local centers and have their materials available. Ask them for suggestions for other materials you can make available to patients.

- *Therapists.* Find local therapists trained *and experienced* in working with sexual trauma, and have their contact information available.

21 Addictions

A wise person should alienate himself from the habitual malpractices gradually. Adoption of good practices should also be in similar way.
CHARAKA[1]

Habit is habit and not to be flung out of the window by any man, but coaxed downstairs a step at a time.
MARK TWAIN

We are all addicted to something. When we consider that everything we do, eat, think, imbibe, or experience alters our chemistry to some extent, we can see that we are all addicted to certain substances and experiences. Some addictions are fairly benign, some even positive, but addictions to alcohol and mind-altering drugs can threaten our health, our relationships, and our jobs, and are frequently fatal. They are also widespread and worthy of serious attention. Since alcohol addiction is by far the most common addiction to mind-altering substances, we will mostly explore this in this chapter, but some of what we explore will certainly apply to other addictions.

Excessive drinking is a major public health problem, and one we will doubtless encounter in a private practice of any significant volume. Excessive drinking results in 88,000 deaths a year, from alcohol poisoning, liver disease, and car or other accidents. In 2006, it cost the US US$223.5 billion.[2] And it causes emotional and physical secondary tolls on relatives of drinkers.

Let us look at the different categories of drinking:

- *Heavy drinking.* If you're a man who has drunk 15 or more drinks per week, or a woman who has drunk eight or more drinks per week, any time in the last 30 days, you would fall into this category.[3] (A standard drink is defined as one 12-ounce bottle of beer, one 5-ounce glass of wine, or 1.5 ounces of distilled spirits.)

- *Binge drinking.* If, within the past 30 days, you are a man and have drunk five or more drinks, or a woman and have drunk four or more drinks, on a single occasion, at least one time, you would be considered a binge drinker. Binge drinkers are at a greater risk than non-binge drinkers, to become dependent. Binge drinking is also associated with many other health and social problems, like violence, new HIV infections, and unintended pregnancies.[4]

- *Excessive drinking.* Excessive drinking is defined as either binge drinking or heavy drinking. Minors (people under the minimum legal drinking age) or pregnant women who drink also fall into this category. About 90 percent of adults who drink excessively report binge drinking.[5]

- *Substance abuse.* Substance abuse indicates drinking or consuming other mind-altering drugs, with poor judgment, but not with the brain disease that accompanies dependence or addiction.

- *Substance dependence, or addiction.* Addictive drinking or alcohol dependence is a clinical diagnosis. It is based on criteria in the *Diagnostic and Statistical Manual of Mental Disorders* (Fourth Edition) (DSM-IV).[6] It is indicated when the patient conforms to at least three of the following seven criteria, in the last 12 months:

  - *Tolerance:* It takes more and more of the drug, over time, to experience the same effect.

  - *Withdrawal symptoms:* When the patient doesn't use the drug, they experience withdrawal symptoms.

○ *Continued use of drug despite harm:* The drug has caused the patient physical or psychological harm.

○ *Loss of control:* The patient takes increasingly more of the drug, over time, or for longer durations.

○ *Attempts to cut down:* Despite conscious attempts to quit or reduce drug use, the patient continues to return to the drug.

○ *Salience:* The patient is obsessed with the drug, spending much time obtaining, consuming, thinking about, or recovering from using it.

○ *Reduced involvement:* The patient has increasingly less interest or involvement in normal social or professional activities, because of the drug.

Why are these drinking categories important? I think, as practitioners, we can feel that addressing addiction effectively is so daunting that we sometimes don't address it at all.

But consider this. Far fewer excessive drinkers than we may assume are actually alcohol-dependent. A government survey and study, conducted between 2009 and 2011, found that about nine out of ten excessive drinkers (that is, 90%!) did not meet the diagnostic criteria for alcohol dependence.[7]

This is clinically important because most non-dependent drinkers may significantly reduce or quit drinking with some relatively simple medical policy strategies and clinical preventive services, without requiring addiction treatment.[8] We will look at Brief Intervention Techniques—one of these strategies—in the "What Can We Do?" section later in this chapter. If we incorporate simple screening techniques and approaches like this in our practices, it could have a huge impact on reducing excessive drinking and preventing addiction. We could, for example, intercept binge drinking before it becomes addiction, as binge drinkers are at greater risk for becoming alcohol-dependent.

My patient Betty's father, Richard, lived with Betty and had been a heavy drinker for 40 years, though he was highly functioning and respected in his community. When Richard's drinking began to cause him to black out and hurt himself on a regular basis, Betty secretly called her father's primary care practitioner who, in the 15 years he had been Richard's doctor, had not once confronted Richard about his drinking. Only when Betty asked him to measure her father's blood alcohol level, and to address the issue, did he do so. He found Richard's blood alcohol significantly elevated. Instead of assessing whether Richard was alcohol-dependent or not, or encouraging Richard to seek treatment for this, or recommending he quit, the doctor told Richard to stop drinking for six months "unless he wanted to die." To Betty's surprise, her father did just that. For six months he did not drink. But on the day the six months were up, he began to drink again, just as heavily as he had before. His doctor never followed up with him about this again, and his addiction took hold firmly again, and ended up causing him great suffering.

The fact that Richard simply quit for six months in response to one simple statement by his doctor demonstrates both the power of the practitioner and the power of a brief statement or "brief intervention." When we overlook or ignore our patients' detrimental habits or addictions, we do them a grave disservice. Literally.

Let us look at alcohol dependence. More than 50 percent of patients struggling with addiction have reported that their primary care practitioner did nothing to address their substance abuse.[9] Many patients will not actively seek help for their addictions. Heroes in Recovery, a website that works to dispel the stigma associated with addiction, states that although 23 million people each year need help for addiction, only 3 million actually seek it.[10]

Many of us have little professional training in how to recognize and treat addiction. It is often beyond the scope of our practice, but, as with sexual abuse, there are some ideas, facts, and resources that may be helpful, both for us and for our patients. While much of what follows is particularly related to patients with alcohol dependence, many of the concepts could be useful for anyone who drinks excessively whose life, job, or relationships are adversely affected by their alcohol use.

For assistance with this topic, in which I have limited experience, I turned to Durga Leela, B.A., founder of Yoga of Recovery, which brings together yoga, Ayurveda, and the Twelve Step principles to work with practitioners and non-practitioners alike.[11]

Especially in some medical practices, we may see addiction on a daily basis. I have a friend, a physician, who is faced multiple times a day with new or returning patients addicted to pills trying to convince him to prescribe more, when he knows there is no medical reason to do so. While my friend may not fall into this reaction, it can be understandable to tire of what may feel like, or actually be, manipulative behavior from patients who are addicted to alcohol or pills, to harden our hearts, and construct immediate, strong, cold boundaries.

When I brought this up with Durga, she responded by asking details about specific patients I had, who had suffered from addictions. She then quickly and accurately guessed the particular difficulties in each of their situations. Her empathy with each of them as distinct and precious human beings with particular challenges increased my own understanding and empathy.

For example, one patient we discussed was Lisa, the nurse who was addicted to pills (see Chapter 10).

Durga observed that were Lisa to admit her addiction to almost anybody in almost any state in the US, she would be subject to professional disciplinary action, and her license would be suspended or revoked. She would almost surely be fired, reducing her prospects of getting another job in her field, lose her status in her community, and lose her dignity. In fact, that is exactly what happened. Eventually Lisa's habit was discovered and she lost her job. Addicts face very real disincentives to even admitting their dependency. One of the largest obstacles in the way of recovery is the derision or punitive response to an addict's behavior or admission. Durga says there can be a tendency to withhold love from the addict until they "learn to behave properly."

Addiction, Durga suggests, is in great measure a disease of isolation. When we respond punitively to an admission of addiction, the addict may retreat again into severe isolation or into the company of people who support or perpetuate the addiction. This is the opposite of healing, and a wasted opportunity to help. If we offer empathy, it may be possible to move forward with the patient's healing.

Many addicts in recovery, say Durga and others, report a moment of clarity and truth[12] that preceded a sudden conversion to recovery. This is a moment where one's vision becomes so clear and powerful that it is life changing, a moment where we realize our addiction is violating our personal values. This moment marks a turning point.

Gabe was an alcoholic and an influential member of his community. He didn't drink publicly. He kept a bottle of high-proof vodka under the seat in his car, and he would only drink there, using his influence to get out of tickets and trouble. One day Gabe was taking a swig out of his bottle while he was driving when he had a premonition that there would be a police car around the next bend. He quickly put his bottle away, and when he reached the bend, sure enough, there was a police cruiser. At that moment, he thought, "This is boring. You have to stop this." That was Gabe's turning point.

The words that Gabe's mind served up for his moment of clarity were, "This is boring." A moment of clarity doesn't have to be awe-inspiring, exciting, or sexy. It just has to show up.

Durga suggests that this moment of clarity is an "internally generated moment of grace," but she allows that there may be "grace carriers," people who will speak to the addict directly, but with empathy. As practitioners, we can't force a moment of clarity on a patient, but we can create a space and cultivate a perspective that invites it.

When the patient feels a break in his isolation, it can be possible to introduce good company, therapy, people, or even literature that may support or accompany the patient on his trek towards a healthier, happier life. Durga pointed out that the metaphorical significance in the difference between "illness" and "wellness" is in how the words begin: "illness" begins with an "i," while "wellness" starts with "we."

My guru once told me, "Keep good company. Good company makes a man great." It can be helpful to remember that service to others is one way to encourage community. I remember years ago hearing a lecture by a man in long-term recovery. He had aided countless people to recovery, and he said that the difference he found between people who could maintain sobriety and those who couldn't was service. People who served others and helped others with their struggle were more successful staying sober. If we can find good company and serve it, it may serve us even more. It may serve to support us as we shift our identity.

Identification (*Ahamkara*)

In Chapter 2, in the section on refining our ability to see, we looked at the Eastern medical premise that *prana*, or life force, follows attention. Let us add to this the concept in Ayurveda called *ahamkara*, literally, the "I former," that defines who we believe ourselves to be. It is what defines our personal identity. *Ahamkara* lines up behind *prana* and attention. We identify with what we focus on, do, and practice. This is why, when what we do is threatened, we may feel personally threatened. If my job, marriage, relationship, addiction, or favorite pastime is taken away, it may not actually be a threat to my person, but I can feel a twist of a knife accompanying these events. Our identity is so intertwined with what we do, that we do not experience ourselves as separate from it. This can be especially true in the case of addiction.

If we have an addiction to a substance, relationship, or habit that is not serving our long-term health, it would be a mistake to try to remove it without first replacing it, because it is a pillar supporting our very identity. What can we replace it with? We can begin by visualizing ourselves without the addiction in a way that we can admire. Often, we don't want to quit something because of what it says about who we are. So we have to create a new image of ourselves that we can visualize and assimilate into the fabric of our being.

If we can visualize it, we can become it. Imagination and action are inseparable. In one study, for example, when people practiced a particular exercise in their imagination, they increased their muscle strength by 22 percent. Those who actually performed the exercise physically gained 30 percent—only 8 percent more than the people who exercised in their imagination.[13]

When I was a teenager, I drank beer. I really enjoyed being the Girl-Who-Brought-the-Beer. I loved being fun-loving. When I considered quitting drinking, one hard part was thinking that I would look like a prude, and lose my fun-loving, Bearer-of-Beer identity. I became committed to stopping, but I still loved my friends and my identity. I steeled myself, and decided that I would bring six-packs of non-alcoholic beer, and make jokes about it. Then my identity might shift a little, but in a way that was attractive to me. I visualized a persona (though that is not how I would have expressed it at the time) that was sufficiently appealing to replace the old one. Identity crisis averted, I quit drinking. And never looked back. I am not saying that it should be this easy for everybody to quit something. I began drinking at around 15 and quit a couple of years later. I do not equate my relatively short-term drinking to more tenacious addictions, but I do think that finding an attractive way to see ourselves sans our bad habits can be a useful tool for change.

Being an empathetic practitioner may help our patients become open to shifting their identity to one that supports sobriety, and to finding good company instead of feeling judged and retreating into the isolation of an addiction.

If we are unable to muster empathy, it is best if we recognize this, refer the patient to someone who can, and address our own limitations in this area when we are able. Somewhere along the way we may have learned that a non-empathetic response is appropriate, or it could be an effect of our own history of association, abuse, and relationships with alcohol or addicts in our lives or families of origin.

If we suspect or know a patient is addicted to a harmful substance, there are a few things we can keep in mind and a few things we can do. The first may be to cultivate empathy. To do this, there are a few things that can help.

What to Keep in Mind to Support Empathy and Guide Our Thinking

When another person makes you suffer, it is because he suffers deeply within himself, and his suffering is spilling over. He does not need punishment; he needs help.
THICH NAHT HANH

- As mentioned before, there are often real obstacles between the patient and recovery that we know nothing about. As in Lisa's case, there may be the fear of rejection, retribution, and punishment.

- The addict's identity is so intimately associated with the use of their chosen substance (or substances), that the thought of giving it up can feel like cutting off an arm. It will be important to coax or support a revised identity—one that aligns with a new reality.

- Many alcohol and drug addicts also suffer from eating disorders or mental illness, and the vast majority of addicts have suffered physical, sexual, or emotional abuse. Many also grew up with eating disorders. Their eating disorder may or may not have a label like bulimia or anorexia nervosa. Even an undue focus on food, portions, calories, or nutrition can cause neurosis around food. Such undue focus may be a kind of neurosis disguised as intelligence. In any case, the complicated history that is closely associated with the addiction may render even simple dietary or lifestyle suggestions emotionally triggering for the patient. This can mean that without at least concurrent professional treatment or therapy for the addiction, the treatment we generally offer may be insufficient. We may go round and round, trying to find an avenue to healing, but discover that each avenue is so obstructed by the addiction that without addressing it directly, we only hit dead ends.

- In Alcoholics Anonymous they say: "Resentment is the 'number one' offender. It destroys more alcoholics than anything else. From it stems all forms of spiritual disease, for we have been not only mentally and physically ill, we have been spiritually sick." While the addict may sound or feel full of resentment and blame, unwilling to shoulder responsibility for his life, he may be willing to point a finger and say, "They did this to me." As the process of identification shifts through the addict's treatment and recovery, it may be easier for him to shift perspective on this. In working with such people, we may experience attempts at manipulation or personal insults, and be tempted to react punitively toward the patient. In these moments, we can cultivate empathy by remembering the element of forgiveness, whether we refer this patient out or not. As the Lord's Prayer says, "Forgive us our trespasses as we forgive those who trespass against us." Don't we all wish for forgiveness?

- An addiction to mind-altering substances may result from the pain of separation from the Divine; it may be a corrupted inclination towards Divine union. This is something many of us feel innately, and it is a view that luminaries like Carl Jung shared.[14] When we become disillusioned with this sometimes violent, unjust, unloving, five-element reality that we experience day after day, it is understandable that some may seek an alternate reality, turning to substances that promise to help us get there.

The addict's internal battle and, for that matter, the internal battle of any excessive drinker, may not be unlike the internal battle of each of us. Who among us cannot empathize with their struggle when we look honestly at our own? In Ayurveda, the word *prajnaparadha* translates as "crime against wisdom." It describes a phenomenon common to most of us. We know better, but do something anyway. This could apply to the obvious addictions like alcohol, cigarettes, pills, and other mind-altering substances, but it also applies to a myriad of subtler obsessive habits like gossiping, eating too many sweets or other unhealthy food, criticizing or envying others, indulging laziness, fueling excess ambition, and so on. When we continually ignore or disobey our internal compass, internal stress, and shame, other difficult emotions build up, creating an unpleasant, sometimes intolerable, life. It is comforting to know that the battle is not just in me; it's in every one of us. I am no longer the lone soldier, charging ahead or succumbing to defeat. If I zoom out and see the battlefield is broad and my comrades many, I see I am not alone, and the camaraderie is comforting.

Rick Silberman, a dear friend, recently wrote me his thoughts on addiction. They included his account of his moment of clarity, and expressed the experience many of us have when we turn to substances to bring us closer to the Divine. Here is what he wrote:

> The root cause of all addiction is the same. It is holding the belief that there is anything (or anyone) outside of ourselves that will somehow relieve our pain—that will somehow make this present moment better. You might be thinking, of course, taking a shot or smoking a joint makes me feel better. If it didn't, I wouldn't do it. Obviously true. But what is the price? What is the net outcome? I think it is this: every time you self-medicate, you reinforce two ideas. The first is that there is some alternate state

of being better than now. The second is that you need a drug to get there. Both of these thoughts deprive you of the opportunity to simply be present, to fully experience things as they really are.

The first time I knew that there was something dramatically amiss in my life was a day in my twenties when I was on a bluff looking at a spectacular sunset and all I could think was, "Boy, this would really be beautiful if only I were stoned." I had come to the point where my sober life barely counted anymore. It was merely a state that I had to endure until I could get high again— the place where the real action was.

The only way to end addiction is to relinquish the belief that there is any substance that will make this moment better, that will fix us, regardless of whether it is heroin, ayahuasca, cannabis, alcohol, or caffeine. We have to make peace with Now.

On the deepest level, it is this belief that we are really addicted to. It is also the most difficult habit to kick. The key is not to forget that the game is to be free and whole just as you are—not to settle for a transient high. No matter how sublime or esoteric your drug experiences are, no matter how present they make you feel, any time you use a substance to get there, you have sent yourself the message that you are not enough. And the more often that you demonstrate to yourself that you are incomplete without [fill in the name of your preferred substance here], the harder it is to stop.[15]

What Can We Do?

While interviewing the patient, there are a few things, ideas, and tools we can consider in dealing with suspected or confirmed excessive drinking or addiction. Some of these may work or apply best to certain addictions, while others will most benefit other situations. Some will apply to all cases.

- *Interview with empathy*, as per the discussion above. How we speak with and counsel patients with addictions is an art. Stephen Rollnick, Ph.D., and William R. Miller, Ph.D., have done much work in this area and have coined the term "Motivational Interviewing." As they define it, "Motivational Interviewing is a directive, client-centered counseling style for eliciting behavior change by helping clients to explore and resolve ambivalence." Information on Motivational Interviewing can be found at www.motivationalinterview.net/clinical/whatismi.html

- *Screening.* Consider screening for excessive drinking and addiction during the initial intake. *Ask how much alcohol the patient drinks, and if it is affecting her relationships.* Whether or not the amount our patient is drinking conforms to the official definition of excessive drinking, if it is affecting her relationships, she could benefit from help. Referring her to professionals trained in counseling in substance abuse could help her change directions. Screening helps quickly identify the severity of substance use and helps connect the patient to the appropriate treatment. We can include a question in our health history forms asking, "Is there a history of addiction or mental illness in your family?" If there is, we can remember that there may be a greater likelihood of the patient having issues around addiction, whether to food, alcohol, or other substances. If we are not sure if excessive drinking is accompanied by dependency or not, we can still employ the Brief Intervention Technique discussed below, but that may well be insufficient if there is dependency.

- *Brief Intervention Technique.*[16] This is a term describing a specific technique we can use to increase a patient's awareness regarding their excessive drinking, and to help motivate them to change. This could be an especially effective tool for excessive drinkers who are not (yet) alcohol-dependent. Unlike traditional acute alcoholism treatment, which may last many weeks or months, brief interventions can be given in a matter of minutes. They can decrease alcohol consumption in a variety of populations by an average of 13–34 percent, and can reduce mortality rates by about 23–26 percent. Brief Intervention Techniques involve making statements or asking a set of questions of patients we believe to have a problem with addiction, especially to alcohol. The simplest brief intervention consists of one or two direct statements: the practitioner tells the patient that her drinking exceeds recommended limits and could lead to alcohol-related problems, and then advises her to reduce the amount she drinks or to stop drinking altogether. (There is a bit more to it than this—information on how to conduct these brief interventions is in the Resources section at the end of this chapter.) Repeated contact with the patient is generally more effective than a single brief intervention. Practitioners can be trained to recognize which patients are most likely to benefit from this technique (not all will), how to conduct brief interventions most effectively, and when it is essential to refer the patient to an addiction specialist. It may sound like this is too simple to work, but remember Richard's story? All it took for him to quit, after drinking excessively for decades, was for his doctor to conduct this kind of brief intervention. Whether or not there is alcohol dependency, we can try this technique. It just may not be sufficient. Also, whether or not there is dependency, we can consider the following points, though they primarily address dependency.

- *Discuss the physical or genetic components of addiction.* From a certain perspective, we could consider addiction a disease of the brain, as the brains of addicts are structurally (and therefore functionally) different from non-addicts, even before a substance is introduced. From another perspective, it could be considered a genetic disorder. Ernest P. Noble, Professor of Psychiatry and Director of the Alcohol Research Center at UCLA's Neuropsychiatric Institute and Hospital, writes that in 1990 researchers linked a gene called DRD2 to severe alcoholism. While only 10 percent of the US population has the A1 variation of the DRD2 gene, it is found in about 50 percent of addicts.[17] Being exposed to scientific or genetic explanations of addiction may help some patients understand why they may be suffering the way they are, and inspire in them the courage to begin recovery. For others, however, it can make them feel even more uncomfortable with, and even betrayed by, their bodies. They may deduce from this that their prospects of recovery are dismal. For these people, appealing to the ego or to the spiritual aspects of the disease may be a more productive and positive approach.

- *Discuss the spiritual nature of addiction.* Durga learned that all disease, including addiction, has a spiritual origin. It all involves forgetting one's true nature as a spark of the Divine. We feel a separation from Truth, from unconditional Love, from the Divine within. We feel disillusioned with this world and its reality, which sometimes seems mad. We long for something meaningful, take solace in the altered perspective that our substance of choice provides us, and miss our calling—our birthright to reunite with the Divine without the aid of mind-altering substances.

- *Appeal to the ego.* The disease of addiction is intimately related to the ego or identification process. The ego is in charge of appearances, and the patient may well wish to keep them up and maintain a certain lifestyle. There are websites and apps like Drinking Mirror that appeal to the ego. You can take your photo (or your patient's photo), plug in how much you drink, and see how you will look in ten years' time if you keep drinking at that rate. These apps are somewhat simplistic, but depending on the nature of the patient and your relationship with her, it might be an effective and light-hearted tool to appeal to her vanity or ego enough to motivate her to change. Many of us feel a need to maintain a face or position in the world. Recognizing that this will get harder the longer they drink or use may help them get into recovery.

- *Re-invent the ego.* One way or another, for recovery to occur, the identification process needs to be rearranged. We need to replace our self-image with something equally or more attractive. One simple tool that might be useful in concert with other treatment (I have also seen it useful in quitting cigarettes) is for the patient to picture himself as someone he respects and admire who *doesn't* use alcohol, cigarettes, or drugs. It is almost impossible to move towards something that repels you. So, if the prospect of being the kind of person who is sober is repellent to us, we won't want to become one. We won't want to identify with one of those puritanical, square, and boring teetotalers. The client can invent an image or picture of a "me" who is attractive without the addiction. He can envision the inner sober person in such a way as to like what he sees. What would this person look like? If, as physicians, we can also focus on seeing the patient's inner sober person, we may be able to help strengthen it.

- *Re-invent the story.* As we saw above, Ayurvedic physician and author Dr. Robert Svoboda said, "The job of the healer is to hear the story and help the person reweave the story." If this is true in general, it may be even more relevant in the case of addicts. As with re-inventing the ego and re-imagining our future self, the same must happen with the story or narrative of the patient's life. The story can change from, "They did this to me," to "I have a brain that is prone to this disease of addiction, but I can find tools to address that." Or "If I want to continue to be successful in my life, relationships, and job, I need to resolve this." Or "Somewhere along the way, my pain of separation from the Divine led me to seek an altered reality, but now I can find tools to help me feel closer to the Divine without this addiction."

- *You don't have to live like this anymore.* Durga says that it can be powerful and effective to look the person in the eye and say with empathy and compassion, if not true understanding, "You don't have to live like this anymore." This will be more powerful if we have fought the same battle, but as human beings unified in part by our ability to empathize even with experiences beyond our ken, it can be effective regardless of the practitioner's personal history.

- *Detach with love.* Offering empathy is not to be confused with enabling a patient to perpetuate unhealthy or abusive behavior, tolerating their manipulation, or allowing inappropriate personal boundaries. We need to employ boundaries, but, as Durga says, while always remembering that the individual is a spark of the Divine. It is good to remember this with everyone of course, not only with addicts. But it can be more challenging to remember it with addicts or other patients with poor personal or emotional boundaries.

- *If someone resists help.* Chapter 11 of the *Su Wen*, a classical Chinese Medicine text, advises, "If one does not accept being treated and cured, do not treat him." We can provide what is in our scope of practice and in our heart to provide. We can provide resources for the patient to take advantage of. We can lovingly detach and then wait. If the patient is not ready, we can do the same and treat what we can or refer the patient to a practitioner who is better matched.

- *Provide resources and referrals to treatment and good company.* We can convey the message, "I recognize you. I see your struggle. And I want you to know that you don't have to live like this anymore. There are compassionate people and organizations that are trained to support your recovery. Here is a list of some of them." We should have a list available.

- *SBIRT: Screening, Brief Intervention, and Referral to Treatment.* SBIRT is one of those mnemonic devices coined to help practitioners remember what to do. Each of its components is addressed above.

Resources

The longer addiction continues, the harder it is to treat. It is progressive and can be fatal. There is no medicine a patient can take to cure his addiction. Its roots may be karmic, spiritual, genetic, or biological. It is a complicated process, and there are professionals and organizations that have been studying and working with addiction and supporting addicts for decades. They can help remove the stigma associated with addiction, and provide good company in one form or another. Many are well trained in addressing the points raised in this section. If we do not feel well trained in these issues, we can refer the patient to someone who is.

Here is a general and incomplete list of resources useful to either practitioner or patient. It would be good to translate this into a list of local branches, when applicable:

- For information about how to conduct brief interventions, see NIH (National Institute on Alcohol Abuse and Alcoholism) (2005) *Helping Patients Who Drink Too Much: A Clinician's*

Guide. NIH Pub. No. 05–3769. Bethesda, MD: NIH. Available at http://pubs.niaaa.nih.gov/publications/AA66/AA66.htm

- The work of Gabor Mate at http://drgabormate.com Dr. Mate shares with great compassion and insight his vast experience with working with addition. This can be useful for both practitioner and patient.

- Alcoholics Anonymous offers free group support and a Twelve Steps program for recovery. It is a source of good company. Participants trade isolation for connection, get a sponsor, and work the Twelve Steps. Working the steps is a process of self-enquiry and self-honesty.

- Therapists who specialize in addiction. Research which professionals in your area have both training and experience in addiction.

- Exercise classes and yoga classes. Exercise can be vitally helpful in the recovery process.

- National Acupuncture Detoxification Association (NADA) (www.acudetox.com). This is a simple, five-needle ear acupuncture protocol that has been proven to reduce the rate of recidivism and support recovery from addiction. It is often offered for free or low cost, and there may be a local treatment center. Their mission statement is: "The National Acupuncture Detoxification Association (NADA), a not-for-profit training and advocacy organization, encourages community wellness through the use of a standardized auricular acupuncture protocol for behavioral health, including addictions, mental health, and disaster and emotional trauma. We work to improve access and effectiveness of care through promoting policies and practices which integrate NADA-style treatment with other Western behavioral health modalities."

- Other Twelve Steps programs, like Al-Anon (for friends and family members of alcoholics) and Narcotics Anonymous, have their own websites and local meetings.

- Yoga of Recovery (http://yogaofrecovery.com), founded by Durga Leela, believes the root cause of addiction is the addict's relationship with self, others, and with God. Yoga of Recovery integrates Ayurveda, yoga, and the tools of Twelve Steps recovery. It offers training for practitioners and people in recovery.

- Genetic links to addiction. If patients are interested in the genetic influences on and associations with alcoholism, they may want to study the work of Ken Blum, a researcher in neuropsychopharmacology and genetics (http://en.wikipedia.org/wiki/Kenneth_Blum).

- Drinking Mirror. This app gives a rather simplistic but possibly effective visual demonstration of how alcohol will affect your looks in ten years' time if you keep on drinking.

- Addressing the stigma and providing a forum for community. Here are a few organizations committed to eliminating the social stigma associated with addiction, and creating active, inspiring, sober communities.

  ○ Heroes in Recovery (www.heroesinrecovery.com/about).

  ○ Erase The Stigma Now (http://erasethestigmanow.com/aboutus.php).

  ○ Faces and Voices Association of Recovery Community Organizations (www.facesandvoicesofrecovery.org/who/arco) is also a forum for uniting and supporting local, regional, and statewide recovery community organizations.

22 Mental Illness

People who suffer from addictions often have some form of associated mental illness. But there are plenty of people with mental illness who are able to avoid addictions that may worsen the condition. In any case, mental illness is rampant in our society and, like addiction, can be fatal. Many forms of CAM address depression, irritability, sadness, and other forms of emotional disequilibrium, but depending on the severity of the mental health disorder of our patient, we may need to refer him to a professional for specialized treatment concurrent with what we can offer.

Along with the helpful perspectives on mental disorders that are taught in many CAM traditions, there are a few things I have learned that have influenced my approach to mental illness, even in its mild forms.

One is the concept of alignment: how aligning with an idea, a representation of the Divine, or even a talisman can help us orient our identities in such a way that we are comfortable participating in life with greater confidence. Shaman Malidoma Patrice Somé, Ph.D.,[1] is an elder of the Dagara people of West Africa, an author, and teacher who has spent a good deal of time considering how mental illness is viewed, understood, and treated in Western countries versus in Africa. In the West, we view a mental disorder as something that needs to stop. Dr. Somé has a different view. He considers mental disorders to be spiritual emergencies of sorts—indications that something from the spirit world is knocking on the door of the consciousness of the patient: mental disorder has arisen because the knocking has been ignored.[2]

Whether or not we believe in spirit realms, we can appreciate the fact that the Dagara people sometimes have more positive outcomes with mental illness than we in the West do.[3] We can also appreciate the underlying principle that, as Dr. Somé says, "Mental disorder, behavioral disorder of all kinds, signal the fact that two obviously incompatible energies have merged into the same field."[4]

I had a patient in his late 30s, who was a large man with an athletic build and deep voice. José looked and acted like a "man's man." He had been on the football team in high school. He now worked as a computer engineer and played basketball in the evenings and weekends. When he came to see me, he was suffering from insomnia, twitching, and panic attacks, and reported feeling like he was "going crazy."

When I asked him about his life, he told me that his grandfather had been a traditional healer in his village in Mexico, and that he himself had very vivid dreams. Sometimes he felt he could "see into the hearts of other people," he said. José could sit for hours at a time, feeling powerful feelings. This had disturbed him for a very long time. He explained, "I am not psychic. I am not the kind of person who should feel these things or think these things." They threatened his identity. They did not fit his sports-loving, beer-drinking, down-to-earth persona. José had embraced Western culture, and considered his grandfather and the old culture backward.

But the discrepancy between how he acted and appeared to the world, and what he was feeling and experiencing inside, was causing José real mental stress and anguish. The cultural context in which he found himself, indeed, which many in the West find themselves, did not recognize sensitivity, spirituality, or psychic phenomenon as practical, valuable, or even authentic aspects of life. Rather, the culture embraced fast-paced living and sensory bombardment, both of which aggravated José's natural pace and triggered a constant background noise of panic.

When we find ourselves unable to fully align with the identity we have formed, when we are haunted by the persistent suggestion that we are somehow more, less, or different than we thought, or that something more is trying to manifest in our lives, we can feel very unstable. We know deep down that our adopted identity is insufficient to embrace our persistent feelings, but change may feel threatening, so we are scared to align with our "new" reality.

Dr. Somé suggests that those of us who find ourselves in this situation need to find something to align with. In this case, in Africa, a shaman may involve the patient in a ritual designed to help her align with the persistent whisperings of her consciousness. The shaman may provide the patient with a physical representation of this alignment—like a rock from a river or a mountain, from whence Dr. Somé says many spirits come. Dr. Somé suggests that the ritual doesn't have to be complicated, and he himself facilitates modified rituals for people in the West.

Whether we think of these persistent whisperings as nature spirits, new influences, or a higher level of sensitivity than our Western culture values, the idea of alignment can be very useful. It may provide a sense of orientation to an identity that may, in turn, offer a sense of comfort and freedom. For José, it was sufficient to bring awareness to the fact that he had been unable to accept what was real for him. He could take an artifact that his grandfather used in his medicine ceremonies and practice, accepting that artifact with respect, rather than resisting it with derision.

When mental illness becomes severe, it can be fatal. WHO tells us that worldwide, approximately 1 million people will commit suicide each year. In addition, even more survive suicide attempts than die from them, and then require medical attention.[5] How can we be alert to the severity of a mental illness that one of our patients is experiencing? While we may not be able to ascertain this definitively, it can help to recognize factors that increase the risk of suicide and ask a few questions.

Here are some of the risk factors[6] we know about:

- History of previous suicide attempts, either of the patient or in the patient's family history.

- History of depression or other mental illness.

- History of alcohol or drug abuse.

- Stressful life event or loss.

- Easy access to lethal methods.

- Exposure to the suicidal behavior of others.

On The Moth podcast,[7] Brian Finkelstein shares some training and wisdom he gleaned from working at a suicide hotline for four years. He was taught that if you are not sure if someone is serious about suicide, there are four questions to ask:

1. Do you ever feel so bad that you think about suicide?

2. Do you have a plan for how you would do it?

3. Have you set a time for when you're going to do it?

4. Have you taken any steps today to kill yourself?

The more "yes" answers, the more critical the situation. Many people would answer "yes" to the first, but "no" to the final three. Aside from these four questions, Finkelstein learned that a big warning sign was when someone says something like, "I don't want to die. I just want the pain to stop."

While I have never had a patient who replied in the affirmative to all four questions, or who said, "I just want the pain to stop," in this context, I feel more assured having an idea of what to listen for. I also appreciate having a way to gauge when someone's mental state is so severely disrupted it may be fatal and immediate assistance is required from someone trained in these matters. I would hate to mistake the signs and miss the opportunity to save a life.

What Can We Do?

As with addiction, mental illness can feel lonely and be incredibly isolating. We are isolated from our healthy self, from others, from a feeling of belonging anywhere and to anything. As practitioners, at least when we are with our patients, we can encourage connection by being connected to ourselves and committed to being present, to listening deeply to the narrative of our patients. Patients with addiction or mental illness—as with most other forms of illness—are likely to benefit more significantly from an ongoing health partnership than from a one-time or short-term treatment strategy.

While there are risk factors for suicide, as we have seen, there are also some resources, habits and behaviors that have a protective effect against it. We can counsel patients whom we believe to be at risk to seek them out and cultivate them. They include:

- Communication skills and training in problem-solving and non-violent conflict resolution.

- Clinical care and treatment for emotional, physical, mental, and substance abuse.

- Effective clinical interventions and support.

- Good company and a sense of community connection.

- Ongoing support from therapeutic healthcare relationships and partnerships.

- Beliefs that discourage suicide and encourage seeking help.

- Offer resources, as listed below.

Resources

Again, resources are important. Here are some that are worth compiling:

- The local suicide hotline. If a patient suffering from depression is in the US, he can call 1-800-273-8255 for the National Suicide Prevention Lifeline, 24/7, to be connected to a skilled, trained counselor in the local area. Whatever problems such patients are dealing with, these people want to help them stay alive.

- Phone numbers for experienced local therapists, counselors, psychologists, psychiatrists, shamans, or other practitioners who specialize in mental health. While a shaman might be a good fit for one patient, a psychiatrist will be a better fit for another. Assisting the patient to find a good match may be the best help we can offer.

- Consider exploring with the patient an idea or representation of the Divine they can align with that will afford them mental stability.

23 Eating Disorders

Although eating disorders are widespread, many of us lack professional training in working with them. In Ayurveda we consider that there are three primary sources of *prana, qi,* or life force. These are air, food, and drink. These three are primal requirements that need to be addressed from the time we take our first breath until we take our last. Because our relationship with food and drink begins so early, it has the potential to color and affect our entire lives.

In infancy, we are tremendously vulnerable to impressions. Everything we taste, everything we ingest, everything we experience, and everything we see makes an impression on us. Neural pathways in our brain form quickly and easily with each impression, and when more than one impression is made at the same time, those concurrently formed pathways bond. This phenomenon is sometimes described as, "what fires together, wires together."

If our feeding experiences in infancy and early childhood are coupled with other experiences, those other experiences have the potential to "wire together" with our relationship to and our experience of food and nourishment for the remainder of our lives. If stress or uncomfortable emotions or experiences were associated with food, we may develop a stubborn and stressful relationship with it and with our bodies.

Because the food we ingest becomes our tissues, organs, and systems, and affects our moods and thoughts, it is true, to some extent, that we are what we eat. If our relationship with food is distorted, our sense of self may become distorted as well, and we may distrust the experience of gaining nourishment, especially through food and drink.

In my experience, I believe the majority of eating disorders I have seen have their roots in early childhood. The people I have seen with the most severe anorexia nervosa, for example, have been highly intelligent, lively people with a deep distrust of food, drink, eating, and drinking from very early on in life.

Because of this, as in the case of addictions, it can be very difficult to give patients with food disorders even very basic recommendations about food. Each avenue we take to work with a patient's food will dead-end until the underlying disorder is addressed. And that disorder may well be better addressed by a practitioner educated, trained, and experienced in eating disorders.

Even if it is appropriate to continue to treat this patient with our own modality, it may be helpful to leave the bulk of discussion about food to professionals trained in eating disorders.

If you can't go in the front door, don't try to break it down. Use a different door, or even a window. If the patient is unable to accept nourishment through food or drink, what form of nourishment might they be more willing to accept?

In Ayurveda, the word *sneha* translates as both "oil" and "love." Oil and love deliver similar physiological effects. This is one reason why people who crave love look for it in doughnuts, cookies, French fries, pizza, or other oily foods. Their bodies and minds experience the oily quality as love. Oil and love are both deeply nourishing. Because oil is so nourishing, patients suffering from eating disorders like anorexia nervosa or bulimia may distrust oil and avoid eating or digesting fatty foods. They become thinner and thinner, and their disorder may prove fatal.

But there are other ways to introduce nourishment to the patient. Though she may be unable to ingest nourishment, including oil, orally, she may be more willing to try something like *abhyanga*, the warm oil, self-massage that is commonly prescribed in Ayurveda.[1] Of course, she may be suspicious that applying oil externally could cause her to gain weight, and need assurance that the oil won't make her fat. (It won't.) Theoretically, if the patient can learn to accept love in this form, it may soften her resistance to nourishment in general.

Performing *abhyanga* every morning with a loving attitude may be especially healing for disorders that find their roots in infancy or early childhood. (We will see why morning might be a good time for this, in Chapter 31.)

Ironically, this approach may also be useful in the case of obesity. In this case, the appropriate external application of oil may deliver the physiological experience of love, thus replacing at least some of the *sneha* that the patient would normally—and unconsciously—try to get from food.

While some forms of eating disorders carry familiar labels like anorexia nervosa, bulimia, or obesity, others may be unfamiliar and unnamed.

There is a phenomenon that seems relatively recent involving tremendous attention to meals and mealtimes for children. When I randomly canvass people in my generation and older, most of them report the following about meals and mealtimes when they were children: they were never given a choice about what they would like to eat for a meal. Meals were served, and you either ate them or not. Choosing to eat or not eat was the only decision a child needed to make.

In the modern world, replete with allergies, food sensitivities, and attention to health, it is understandable that more attention might be paid to meal times, but maybe we are going overboard. When we ask the child what he would like for dinner, make him special meals, and then fight with him to get each morsel down his gullet, we may be bundling the experience of nourishment with stress and unnecessary emotion. After all, because young children lack full prefrontal cortex activity, when we ask them to make decisions about food, they will make emotional decisions instead of rational ones. Later in life, this early-formed pattern may encourage emotional eating, stress, and excessive fixation about otherwise healthy eating—a condition recently named orthorexia nervosa.

What Can We Do?

As with other disorders we've explored, it is not the intention of this book to go into depth about understanding and treating eating disorders. But as with those other disorders, there are a few things that can be helpful to keep in mind:

- If the patient will not welcome food as a form of nourishment, consider other forms of nourishment, like warm oil massage, sweet music, or good company. Once the patient is able to accept these other types of nourishment, it may be easier for her to develop trust in food.

- Get a professional on board who is trained in working with the type of eating disorder from which the patient suffers.

- Concurrently with professional help, treat the patient with the tools in our own modalities.

- Provide resources, as listed below.

Resources

- *Therapists.* Find local therapists trained and experienced in working with eating disorders, and have their contact information available.

- *Books.* One that Durga recommends is *Eating in the Light of the Moon: How Women Can Transform Their Relationship with Food Through Myths, Metaphors, and Storytelling,* by Anita Johnston, Carlsbad, CA: Gürze Books, 2000.

- *Eat Breathe Thrive*™ (www.eatbreathethrive.org) is a non-profit program that offers evidence-based programs that integrate yoga and community to support recovery from eating disorders and negative body image.

24

Domestic Violence

Like sexual abuse, this topic could be a book in itself, and practitioners may choose to receive extra training in this area, but in the absence of that, there are at least a few things that are useful to consider.

As with cases of rape and other forms of sexual abuse, ignorant questions abound when it comes to domestic violence, and they are all too easy to ask. Before becoming more educated on the realities of domestic abuse or battering, I myself asked my patients some version of the No. 1 ignorant question: "Why on earth don't you leave him?" (Though I am aware that domestic abusers can be women, I am using the pronoun "him" because far more men than women are perpetrators of domestic violence.) It is one thing to sincerely strive to learn about the real barriers and reasons why a woman doesn't leave an abusive partner. It is another to think it is as easy as walking out the door and to suggest that the woman is weak or ignorant if she doesn't just do it.

There can be many very good reasons a woman will not leave a boyfriend, partner, or husband who is physically or sexually abusive. This woman, passive though she may appear, is an expert on her situation, and she is guaranteed to have thought about those reasons more than her doctor.

Jackie was a long-term patient who had been with a boyfriend who, she reported, used to regularly beat her. He had stopped because he knew he had power over her. He knew she wouldn't leave him. Jackie and I spoke about this openly. I had posted the phone numbers of domestic violence shelter helplines and information in the bathroom of my office, and Jackie knew all about our local resources. She had decided not to avail herself of any of them. At least not yet. She had a grown son in college and an elderly mother in an assisted living facility. She was confident that her boyfriend would injure or kill one or both of them if she were to leave him. She would have had to move an elderly, frail mother and a son to a secret place, somewhere the boyfriend couldn't find. The obstacles to leaving were too great. She decided to bide her time. She felt this was her cross to bear, and her decision alone.

Jackie was grateful for the understanding that nobody could have thought more about her situation than she. To ask her, "Why don't you leave him?" in a tone reflecting incredulity that any woman would put up with this treatment would have simply reflected ignorance of the complexity of her situation, and disrespect of the thoughtful, if difficult, decision Jackie had made. Then she would have felt judged as well as trapped.

We cannot all be trained in everything. Extensive training in domestic violence may not be feasible for all practitioners, but there are a few things we can incorporate into our practices that help afford respect and dignity to people suffering at the hands of an abuser.

With each initial intake, we can gently ask our patient this direct question: "Is anyone hurting you emotionally or physically?" This provides an invitation to provide information that may have tremendous bearing on the wellbeing and prognosis of the patient. If this question is not asked directly, it may be too hard for someone to find the right moment to share this important information.

The patient may, of course, choose to answer truthfully or not, but at least she has an opening if she needs and wants help. I usually preface this question with something like, "This question may sound strange, but it is a question I am committed to asking every patient." And I pretty much am. Unless there is a good reason not to ask this question, I would ask it. I would ask it if the patient was a man or a woman, young or old, rich or poor. I have had patients from all these categories answer in the affirmative.

One spirited elderly woman patient answered me in the affirmative, and when her husband passed away a couple years later and she was decidedly not sorry, I understood. When I asked her my questions, she had been relieved to be honest about it. Another woman was reluctant to answer, but after several treatments, she volunteered her story. She had moved across the country to a gated home that was alarmed to the hilt, and changed her name in order to escape her abuser.

Many patients used this question as a springboard to offer other information. A man would say, "No, not physically, but I feel emotionally battered by my boss." A young woman would answer, "No, but my brother has been a real jerk lately," and go on to describe fairly common, if unpleasant, sibling rivalry. The question does not always reveal serious abuse, but it sends a message that if they are in trouble, you might be able to offer assistance.

Abusers typically exhibit very controlling behavior, and may follow or accompany the person everywhere they go, even to doctor's appointments. They may try to be present during the consultation. Whether or not you suspect abuse, it is possible to say to anyone who has accompanied the patient, "I always conduct this part of the consultation privately. I would like to ask you to sit in the waiting room until I am through." Perhaps you can do this when you begin the part of the intake that addresses gynecological issues, or urogenital issues if the patient is a man. Then you can take that opportunity to ask the question.

In one of the workshops I attended on domestic violence, a middle-aged woman spoke about the first time she told anyone about the abuse she suffered. She was at her doctor's office and was to give blood for some test. When she rolled up her sleeve, he saw severe bruises on her arm. He asked her how she got them. She looked at him, mustered her courage, and told him she was a battered woman. That doctor had many choices in that moment. What he chose to say was, "Well then, we will have to use the vein on the other arm."

She left that doctor's office feeling more hopeless than ever.

It is very possible that a patient, if she feels safe, may choose to confide in her practitioner, even if that practitioner is not trained in helping victims of violence.

Without training in domestic violence counseling or services, what we can offer, aside from kindness and whatever is in our scope of practice, is information. Information can help enormously to connect patients with helpful resources. We can provide domestic violence information, including shelter information and hotline numbers. We can make it a habit to keep a pile of business cards with shelter hotline numbers in the bathroom as well as in our files, so someone can pocket a card in private if they prefer.

Why is it helpful to know if there is domestic violence now occurring, when we may not need confirmation of a history of sexual abuse? Because it could be a life-threatening situation. One way to guess how critical the situation is, is to be aware that there is usually a cycle of violence that goes like this: there is a violent incident, followed by a honeymoon phase where the perpetrator will send flowers, apologize, promise never to do it again, and be relatively well-behaved. Then stress and tension build. Then there is another incident of violence. This cycle repeats itself. If the cycles get shorter, the danger is growing. For example, if the perpetrator used to injure the patient once a year or so, and now it is more like once a month, the chance of a mortal incident is increased.

To best support patients who suffer at the hands of an abuser, we can receive training in this ourselves, or offer good resources.

What Can We Do?

- Make it a policy to ask every patient, "Is anybody hurting you, emotionally or physically?"

- Refrain from asking, "Why don't you leave him?" with judgment. This implies that the patient is ignorant, weak, or careless of her situation. She may have compelling reasons to stay.

- Receive training in domestic violence issues.

- Provide resources, like those below.

Resources

- *Domestic violence shelters.* Most cities have resources for victims of domestic violence. If there is a domestic violence shelter or hotline in your area, they are likely to know what resources are available, as well as being a resource themselves. Keep a stack of business cards with domestic violence shelter and hotline numbers in your office bathroom, as well as your front office. This way, if a patient does not want to disclose abuse, there is a confidential way they can still access resources.

- *Therapists.* Find local therapists trained and experienced in working with domestic abuse, and have their contact information available.

25 Determining the Severity of a Crisis

There are two types of persons having misleading appearance. One is the person who, though suffering from a severe disease, appears to be suffering from a mild disease, because of the excellence of physical and emotional stability and strength. The other is a person who, though suffering from a mild disorder, appears to be suffering from a severe disorder because of a weak physical or emotional constitution. Physicians who are not acquainted with these two deceptive appearances fail to decide mildness or severity of a disease, proceeding only on gross observation of the patient.
CHARAKA[1]

You should not burden your mind with anxieties about [your patients]. Keep your mind free. Your treatment and service will help them, but not your worrying about them. Worry weakens your power to be useful to them.
SAWAN SINGH JI MAHARAJ[2]

I was at a yoga retreat with a long-time friend. While there, one of the participants in a very gentle restorative yoga class—let's call her Susan—began to writhe on the floor, exclaiming about a terrible pain she said was caused by simply raising her arms over her head. She didn't focus her eyes on anyone else's, and seemed consumed with her own need.

Three of us—the very experienced yoga instructor, a chiropractor who happened to be in the class, and I—took her aside, assessed her, and could not find anything wrong with her physically. Telling her this, however, would not have worked, as she would have felt that we weren't respectful of her assessment. Susan was crying for validation of her pain, which appeared largely emotional. She was almost demanding to go to the hospital, but it was clear to the professionals there that a trip to the hospital might make her more scared and would be unproductive, since there was nothing physically wrong with her. In the end, we provided a very, very simple treatment for anxiety, but named and explained it in Eastern medical terms, so she was reassured that there was indeed a problem, and it could be named and treated. Comforted by this and by the attention she received, Susan was fine within an hour or so. Then we were able to gently provide her with resources for her ongoing mental and physical health. Although Susan was convinced her crisis was physical, it was more likely a crisis of mental health or a result of an addiction to a substance we weren't aware of.

In the opposite case, I have had patients who ignored very real pain that was heralding serious health concerns, thinking the pain would pass and probably wasn't serious. These are people who have too great a tolerance for pain and risk serious repercussions to their health by ignoring their symptoms.

As practitioners, staying centered puts us in a better position to come to our own conclusions about our patients' conditions and not to respond reactively to their assessments. Patients may be clear about their own feelings—physical and emotional. But just as a valley dweller has a different perspective than someone who lives on top of a mountain, a practitioner has a different perspective on a client's pain—as long as she does not identify too closely with it. Remember, too, that Charaka counsels us not to rely on the testimony of an addict or someone attached to a particular outcome.

A patient's emotional crisis should not become our emotional crisis. Empathy is good, but over-identification with the patient's feelings may cause us to lose a helpful perspective. To keep a steady head and hand, we can step back and assess for ourselves if there is need for immediate referral to professional mental or physical emergency care. Then we can respond accordingly. Swift action may indeed be required, but sometimes we can discern when the crisis is more in the patient's perspective than physical reality.

It is not uncommon for people suffering from great anxiety, depression, or instability to believe there is a threat to their physical health or mortality. The intensity of their conviction may be convincing to those close to them, especially if they are not trained in medicine. Staying steady, assessing the situation, referring to specialists immediately if necessary, and otherwise treating the condition that we ourselves assess can lend calmness to an otherwise potentially unstable situation.

What Can We Do?

If we are not sure if something is a crisis, there are a few things we can do, in this order:

- Assess, to the best of our ability, if there is a physical condition that warrants immediate referral to professionals trained to respond to physical emergencies. Usually the emergency room is an appropriate referral in this case.

- Assess, to the best of our ability, if there is a mental condition that warrants immediate referral to professionals trained to respond to mental health emergencies. *Have these phone numbers readily available.*

- If you are not sure if what you are seeing is a crisis or not, you can call 911 (or whatever is your emergency service contact in your country of practice) and defer to their judgment. The worst that can happen if you do is you inconvenience people. The worst that can happen if you don't is the patient could die.

- If the patient is emotionally upset but not in need of immediate mental healthcare, it is still likely she would benefit from referral to a mental health professional. If appropriate, we can concurrently and calmly treat them—if they want us to—in whatever modality we work.

26 Telephone Availability and Crisis

I had been in practice for about three years, and I rarely felt shocked by patients' revelations or conditions. I felt sturdy. Then one evening, I received a phone message from Jane. She was crying hysterically and "joking" through her tears about the ways she could kill herself.

This may have been less dramatic than some of the things I had encountered in my practice, but in the amount of time it took to listen to Jane's message, I felt shaken to my core.

I received probably a dozen or so emotionally dramatic phone messages over the course of my private practice. These are messages of emotional crisis, either due to mental or emotional disorders or to issues surrounding addiction. Phone messages can feel very intrusive. What may not shock us in person, in a clinical setting where we are prepared and have resources at our fingertips, may shock us on a phone message or an email we get in our own home, car, or other personal space. When a patient is not present to see our body language and receive immediate feedback, he may feel free to more fully unpack his grief or anger, beyond what is appropriate, thus passing the buck to his practitioner.

In studies of stress responses in rats, it has been found that when rats take out their frustration on other rats—by chewing on or otherwise bullying them—they transfer their frustration to those rats, thereby lowering their own stress level. This may be a human coping mechanism, too. A more benign interpretation is that it is a natural human instinct to pick up the phone and connect with someone we trust when we are in crisis.

Picking up the phone, calling a friend or a doctor and screaming, may help the patient feel a little better, but it can be disturbing for the unsuspecting recipient. It is not that I do not have empathy for people in emotional crisis. It is that I am not an emergency healthcare worker. Professionals trained to manage crisis are generally better equipped to deal with this sort of emergency. Unless we are trained in this sort of crisis management and wish to work with this population, it is worth figuring out who is, and making their hotline numbers available to people with acute and severe emotional suffering.

What Can We Do?

Along these lines, here are a couple of practical steps we can take:

- Only give out personal contact information to patients fully trusted not to misuse it.

- Have the office outgoing work message say, "If you are having an emergency, please hang up and dial 911." This covers both physical and emotional emergencies.

- Be honest with ourselves about our professional, personal, and emotional limitations, and set policies that reflect them. Our limitations may also change over time. For example, I might make myself more available at times when I have fewer family or other obligations, or after receiving more training in a particular area of crisis management. And I may make myself less available in certain situations—like during family emergencies, if I feel ill equipped to handle a particular kind of crisis, when I am more busy than usual, or when I feel emotionally or physically depleted myself.

- Keep a list of contact information and hotline numbers for professionals or centers trained or specializing in psychiatric care, addiction, suicidal tendencies, domestic violence, etc.

Having these resources at hand is comforting, both for the practitioner and the patient. I may not be able to help the person myself, but it may still comfort her to be given access to people who can.

27 Reflections on Part II

My friend and colleague Edward Kentish, L.Ac., was taught that when you graduate from medical school of any kind, you have a kind of grace period where the Divine will do your work for you. But you should be paying close attention anyway because, when the grace period ends, you will have to do the work yourself, and you will need to know what to do.

I don't know that there is ever a grace period or, if there is one, that it ever ends. But it does seem that confidence is built over time, as a side effect of applying excellence in theoretical knowledge to extensive practical experience. If we see our patients have good results over and over, our confidence grows.

If the pursuit of knowledge yields humility, confidence, improved communication, empathy, the ability to diagnose accurately, and a better outcome for our patients, all these skills and qualities are refined through practicing directly with patients day after day, year after year.

When I talk about our confidence growing, I don't necessarily mean confidence that a certain remedy or therapy will work, but confidence in our ability to see the next right step. Confidence in the fact that even without knowing all that we think we should in an ideal world, our patients get better and we help them do so. We also grow our confidence in the potential for transformation—seeing that when we are patient and allow space and time, there is a power that seems to be ever at the ready to aid it. We develop confidence in the efficacy of simple remedies, in our technical abilities like pulse taking, and in navigating relationships with patients, our environment, and our colleagues. We also gain confidence in discerning when we are in over our heads, and in supporting patients in finding what they need. We develop confidence in our ability to find hope—to find the good. For me, perhaps most importantly, I found I gained confidence in Forces Greater Than Myself.

Humility is refined as we are reminded over and over of what we don't know. It is humbling when treatment outcomes are poor, and perhaps even more humbling when we see seemingly miraculous outcomes. The responsibility of our relationships with our patients is humbling. Spending time at the altar of medicine is humbling.

Our ability to communicate and to empathize is refined as we practice refining our senses, with our patients, over and over and over. Our ability to diagnose is refined through the practice of all these qualities and, as a result, our patients' outcomes are likely improved, as is our ability to practice the art of medicine.

PART **III**

Dexterity

The Value of Flexible Medicine

Discussion with specialists promotes the pursuit and advancement of knowledge, provides dexterity...and creates confidence.
CHARAKA[1]

One day, long after I had begun my medical practice, I was revisiting Charaka's four-part prescription for a decent physician. I understood the need to pursue knowledge and purity, and to acquire practical experience, but...*dexterity*? Why was dexterity important? What did he mean? Was it even a good translation?

I asked my friend, Frederick M. Smith, Ph.D., Professor of Sanskrit and Classical Indian Religions at Iowa University, who assured me that it was.[2] The more I reflected on this word, the more I realized that it is employed a lot in the practice and art of medicine, at its best. Dexterity indicates flexibility with and a facility for different approaches, perspectives, or therapeutic tools. When one thing doesn't work, try another. This is a facility a physician may need to employ on a daily basis, and it can be the determining factor in how often treatment is successful.

28 Reaching Beyond Our Own Field

For explanations of truths and principles quoted from other
branches (of science or philosophy) and incidentally discussed
in the present work, the student is referred to expositions
made by the masters (of those sciences or philosophies),
since it is impossible to deal with all branches of science,
etc. in a single book (and within so short a compass).

By the study of a single shastra, a man can never catch the true
import of this (science of medicine). Therefore, a physician should
study as many allied branches (of science or philosophy) as possible.
The physician who studies the science of medicine from the lips
of his preceptor, and practices medicine after having acquired
experience in his art by constant practice, is the true physician, while
any other man dabbling in the art should be considered an impostor.
SUSHRUTA[1]

While it is clearly not appropriate to practice a form of medicine we
are not trained in, it can be beneficial to learn enough of another
field that we become more dexterous in our own.

Sometimes practitioners think that, not only should they not
stray from their own tradition, but it is also not right even to mix
herbs of different medical traditions. In truth, there is no such
thing as "an Ayurvedic herb," or a "Chinese herb," or any herb that
belongs exclusively to any tradition. There are simply plants and

foods available anywhere that can be analyzed or considered using principles of Ayurveda, TCM, Western herbology, or other traditions. To reach beyond our field and apply our principles to herbs across the globe or in our back yard is not so much breaking the rules as applying dexterity. It also may be helpful for the planet. If we don't have to transport herbs across the globe in order to satisfy our pharmacies, we rely less on fossil fuels, and are more able to ensure that our herbs are grown properly—more about what that might look like in Part VI.

Along with using herbal remedies from various traditions, we may find learning other subjects beneficial. In addition to aspects of modalities outside our own, incorporating philosophies, music, poetry, or art into our practice may increase our dexterity, and therefore improve the chances of a good outcome. Whereas a pill and a lifestyle or dietary change may act as medicine, it may be that a story, a song, or a new way of looking at life or its components is even more effective medicine, and one with fewer side effects.

One malady may be understood elegantly using one explanation or pattern, while another malady may be better explained by a different medical system altogether. For example, one pattern might be most elegantly described using the doshic theory of Ayurveda; another might be better explained using Zang Fu theory in TCM. Similarly, it might be difficult to explain or diagnose a certain condition with either TCM or Ayurveda, but it can be clearly explained using Jyotisha—an astrology practice of India. It is often the case that if we can arrive at an elegant way of understanding or explaining a malady, we may treat it more effectively.

Tom suffered a stroke. There are extensive acupuncture programs recommended for stroke recovery, but he was unable to tolerate strong or too frequent treatments, and I was not in a position to offer as many treatments as he appeared to need, even if he could have tolerated them. But it was possible to find something that he *could* afford and tolerate. He could, for example, use a mirror box on his own to encourage his healing. A mirror box is a relatively new and often effective therapy for stroke rehabilitation, and while not technically within the treatment modalities I practiced, it was easy— both for Tom and me—to learn the basic concepts and incorporate it into a treatment protocol that relied on his efforts more than mine.

Tanya had been a patient for a few years. She would come regularly for support to resolve anxiety and address the occasional symptom or malady. She would have acupuncture and herbs, to which she responded well and quickly. One day she came in with a virulent vaginal yeast infection. She responded quickly to acupuncture and herbs, but when she stopped taking the herbs, the infection returned within a few days. She tried Western medicine, but with the same result. Tanya was doing nothing different in her life or diet. So I turned to Jyotisha. I looked at her chart and saw some astrological influences that had been initiated about the time her infection had begun, and those influences were going to be strong for another nine months. I shared this with her, and together we considered it might be beneficial for her to stay on some herbal remedy for the duration of these influences. And that is exactly what happened. Tanya was able to keep the yeast infection under control for that period of time, and after the influences passed, so did her malady.

We can apply this thinking to the use of subtle medicines like homeopathy, flower remedies, and Reiki, or even the placebo effect, as opposed to the grosser forms of medicine like surgery, drugs, or our beloved herbal remedies. (I am not equating the former forms of medicine with placebos; it is just that they are all subtle—if powerful—forms of medicine.) Just as a hypnotist can learn to recognize which people will be more likely to be receptive to hypnosis, we may be able to consider who would be most likely to benefit from subtle medicine versus gross medicine.

Suppose, for example, we find that placebos work on 30 percent of patients. This tells us something, but perhaps we would learn more if we considered what, if anything, those 30 percent have in common. Or perhaps 90 percent of the people who benefit most from a placebo share certain attributes. If we know this, placebos become a much more powerful form of a medicine, as we can then target those who are more susceptible to them and save the bigger guns—the grosser forms of medicine—for other patients.

For example, I have found that patients who suffer more from anxiety and insomnia, who have delicate constitutions, and who also have more introverted and imaginative emotional and mental profiles seem to respond better to subtler forms of medicine. Patients who are either dominantly intellectual or who have very sturdy, hardy constitutions often do better with education or the grosser medicines, respectively.

When one approach doesn't work, make sense, or resonate, it can be useful to look around and consider what else might work, make sense, or resonate.

29

When the Front Door Is Locked, Use the Back Door, or Even a Window

In healing, one must enquire closely as to the state of the patient's elimination, differentiate the pulse patterns, and observe accurately the patient's emotional, psychological, and spiritual states and other physical manifestations. If a patient is superstitious and does not believe in medicine, or if a patient refuses to be treated by acupuncture, or if a patient refuses any treatment, then no matter what the practitioner does, the patient will not get well. This is evidence that healing actually comes from within.
HUANG DI NEI JING[1]

One man's medicine is another man's poison. What theoretically should work—and practically speaking does work for most people—might worsen someone else's condition. It can be a challenge to find a medicine, protocol, or remedy that a patient can fully embrace.

David, a dear friend of mine, had lived his 68 years with very little stress, high integrity, a lot of joy, a decent diet, and good physical exercise when his heart began to fail for seemingly no reason and with none of the usual precursors. He was told it was a fatal condition.

We considered which medicines and recourses to take. There were complex Ayurvedic and TCM formulas, as well as expensive neutraceuticals that were reported to have promise. David didn't like the idea of most of these and, when he tried them, could not tolerate them. This was a man who had almost never been to a Western medical doctor, lived off the grid in the middle of woodland areas, lived off the land, and always found the cheapest way to do what he wanted to do and fix what needed fixing with materials and resources he had on hand or could easily acquire. I considered which of the mainly local herbal remedies might help his heart and appeal to his sensibility and philosophical outlook. He was able to tolerate these, at least for six months or so, and while his heart condition did end up being fatal, it is possible that the medicines he could tolerate gave him some comfort. What is clear is that the medicines that were most clearly indicated were ones he could not tolerate at all.

If the front door is bolted, try the back door. Or the window. It may not be as easy, quick, or convenient as an unlocked front door, but in the end, it can accomplish the same goal and be more effective than trying to force the front door—that is, push our own agenda.

This happens regularly in a therapeutic relationship. Perhaps the doctor thinks a certain herb or remedy is necessary, and the patient disagrees. Perhaps the doctor thinks a patient's health would improve if he stopped running so much, drinking so much, eating so much, or working so hard, and the patient disagrees.

Nancy came to my practice for treatment for pain between her shoulder blades. I had treated probably hundreds of patients with success with cupping, a remarkably effective therapeutic tool. I was certain it was the best therapy for Nancy.

I explained to Nancy that, while cupping may feel uncomfortable and would likely leave bruise-like marks that would last about a week, I enthusiastically championed this therapy for her. She was resistant to the treatment, and I made this mistake: I trusted my own historical experience over my *current* experience of reality—that is, Nancy's definite resistance.

In the end, Nancy reluctantly agreed to the treatment, and left the office with the promised bruising but without incident otherwise. I noticed later that she had canceled her follow-up treatment. Normally I wouldn't call a patient who had canceled, but something inside me prompted me to check in with her. Nancy told me that since I asked, she had been abused as a child and experienced a devastating loss of control. Agreeing to the cupping, which she had not really wanted to do, had felt re-traumatizing to her. She had left my office having revisited that childhood trauma. She did not make another appointment.

I apologized to Nancy and felt deep remorse about the situation. It was a powerful lesson in the importance of dexterity. Dexterity is a good companion to confidence. I was confident that cupping had the potential to successfully treat Nancy's physical pain. I pushed my own agenda and we both suffered the consequences. Had I deferred to Nancy's reluctance, I could have found more gentle ways to address her physical pain without aggravating her emotional discomfort. It might have taken longer to resolve the pain, but it could have been a welcomed and ultimately effective treatment.

I have found that welcomed treatment is significantly more harmonious and effective than distrusted treatment. Indeed, if a patient is resistant, the resistance may translate physically as complications or even a worsening of symptoms.

When I see or feel a patient truly welcome a treatment or therapy with open arms and heart, I find it a powerful augury of a good outcome.

30

When Patients Consistently Experience Odd Reactions to Remedies

Another situation in which we can apply dexterity is with patients who don't respond to remedies the way we expect, based on theory and our experience.

When I was first in a busy practice, around 1997, I found that roughly 1 percent of my patients (this is an estimate) responded to herbs or remedies in an unpredictable way. Let's say I gave someone a laxative herb that was effective in the vast majority of my patients. Not only would it prove ineffective, but the patient would also react to it with some obscure symptom, like a shooting pain in their second left toe.

I found that with this subset of patients there had often been clues that they were highly sensitive. The main "clue" was that many of these patients already knew this about themselves and announced it. Whenever someone told me they were generally more sensitive to remedies, or had strange reactions to them, they probably were and did.

If someone reacts unusually to one remedy, they may also react unusually to others. For example, if someone was particularly sensitive to touch or needles, I would consider it more likely that they would also be extra sensitive to herbal remedies. In these cases, I found it usually best to offer one or *maybe* two simple remedies, lifestyle, or dietary changes, and to do so only after seeing that the person really embraced the proposed remedy or change. Together we would find a strategy they could embrace, and watch as they implemented that change to confirm things were moving in the right direction.

It seems to me that the percentage of patients that experience a heightened sensitivity to remedies has been growing. If it was about 1 percent when I was first in practice, I think I would now estimate 5–10 percent. In any case, if we are in a busy practice, we will encounter this and it is worthwhile to have an approach ready to address it.

31 Loopholes
Thinking Outside the Box

One of my favorite themes in India is that of loopholes. Here's an example. To be a good Hindu, it is said that you should visit X number of important pilgrimage sites throughout India in your lifetime. If you can't do that, it will suffice to travel to a smaller number of specific holy sites. If you can't manage that, you can just do the *panchakroshi yatra*, which encircles Benares, visiting X number of temples along that path. If you are unable to visit all of those, you can visit a smaller number. If that is still beyond your means, you can go to the three main pilgrimage sites in Benares. And if you can't do that, you can just go to one: *manikarnika ghat*. If even that is beyond what you are capable of, then if you just visualize *manikarnika ghat* once a day, from wherever you are, you are a good Hindu.

Even if I got the details wrong in this example (and I am reasonably confident that I did), you get the idea. There is always hope. If you can't do the ideal, you can get as close to it as you can and, if you do that with sincerity, it will still be acceptable. This always reminds me of the woman whose small donation counted more to Jesus than the larger donation from the rich man because the woman was giving something when she could afford nothing, and she did it with love and sincerity. And it counted.

If the usual practical and scientifically "proven" methods of treatment don't work, we are forced to think outside the box: to experiment, to theorize, to work with our patients to come up with something unique—something that appeals to them, to their understanding of reality, sensibility, and nature. Such experiments are hardly ones we might trot out for scrutiny, as we are doing something new and unproven. But when we consider that even the most scientifically proven medications are an experiment when applied to an individual patient, we have to acknowledge that we are *all* great experiments. Creative solutions can be well worth trying.

If we can't treat something in an obvious way (and really, even if we can), we can look for loopholes that make treatment more effective or offer a solution when nothing else seems to fit as well. One of my favorite loopholes is the idea that each human being is a microcosm of the macrocosm.

Microcosm and Macrocosm

> The individual is not different from the universe. All natural phenomenon in the universe exist in the individual. The wise desire to perceive all phenomena in this way.
> CHARAKA[1]

The Eastern concept of microcosm and macrocosm states that the natural phenomena we find in the universe also exist in the individual, and vice versa.

If we apply this idea to temporal cycles within the universe and in the lifetime of a human being, we can see a pattern. For example, in a yearly cycle, cold, dark seasons give way to lighter, warmer, more active seasons, which eventually return again to cold, darker winter months. Similarly, daytime is born from, and yields to, night-time in the daily 24 hours cycles. Correspondingly, man is born from the darkness of the womb, into the light, active daylight of a lifetime, and eventually succumbs to the quieting of old age and death. For our purposes, let us consider specifically the daily cycle in relation to a human lifespan.

We know that that the musical note C revisits itself again and again, going up or down the scale in various octaves. Similarly, archetypal experiences repeat in each temporal cycle: birth and dawn represent beginnings and change; midlife and midday represent heightened activity; and death and nightfall represent endings and transitions.

Because the latter in each pair is a microcosm of the former, when we affect one, we affect the other.

How is this a loophole? Let's say we are having trouble treating imbalances related to one of these three stages of life—early, middle, or late. We could try to maximize the effects of treatment by administering it at the corresponding time of day. We could consider whether a disorder is most related to issues stemming from a difficult birth or childhood, from imbalances in the ambitious years of raising a family and engaging in a profession, or from issues mostly related to old age. If there is a specific stage of life from which a disorder has arisen, we can prescribe remedies, actions, visualizations, or habits that the patient can incorporate, take, or practice during the corresponding part of the day.

I've applied this theory most often to the correlation between birth and dawn. It is very common to see patients who have suffered from physical, emotional, or mental disorders since childhood. The language they use in these cases runs along the lines of, "I have suffered from this as long as I can remember," or "Since my childhood...", or "This is the way I have always been."

When there is this kind of profile, it is possible that this person's disorder was caused by stress or trauma in utero, during birth, or in early childhood. Often she feels a sense of hopelessness about changing these patterns. Indeed, Ayurveda and many other medical modalities recognize that when we suffer in the developmental stage of our life, those impressions are so tenacious that they are sometimes considered permanent. For example, a fetus affected by its mother's alcohol or drug consumption may have lifelong disorders to contend with.

The idea that such maladies are permanent troubled me. If true, it meant that something we had no control over as a developing fetus, infant, or young child could limit us for the rest of our lives—negatively impacting our ability to have intimate relationships, trust others, or digest physical or emotional experiences.

I was particularly troubled by this because my guru had told me that a doctor should *always* think that he will be able to find "the cure of the pain of the person." He didn't say there were certain conditions that were hopeless. He told me that the outcome of a treatment was not in my hands—it was in the hands of God—but that it is the job of both doctors and patients to make sincere efforts. How was I to feel optimistic about people suffering from such tenacious and lifelong maladies?

I looked for a loophole. When I considered this temporal one, I began to apply it.

I had traveled to another state and consulted with some new patients there. Elizabeth was one of them, and she came in with a list of disorders. Three of the most tenacious and bothersome complaints had been with her as long as she could remember. It seemed to me that many of her other complaints would likely clear up if these three issues could resolve.

Over the course of our conversation, I had a strong feeling that Elizabeth thought I was a quack. I wondered how she had found her way to see me. Perhaps she had been talked into it by some persuasive friend, but now doubted that decision. I felt I had very little mandate: she probably would not be receptive to a list of lifestyle and diet "dos" and "don'ts." I decided to offer a single remedy. The fact that this remedy might sound crazy to Elizabeth was okay, since she probably already thought I was a bit of a nut.

All three of her major long-standing complaints related most to one of the meridians that forms earliest in fetal development, which indicated the possibility of some trauma there. There are a couple of acupuncture points that "open" that meridian. I suggested that Elizabeth awaken every day at dawn, get in a loving mood, and apply soothing oil to these two acupuncture points, which she could use as acupressure points.

She looked at me like I had two heads. I thought I would likely not hear from her again. I was quite surprised then, when about six months later, I received a note from Elizabeth, telling me that not only had her three lifelong complaints resolved, but many of her minor complaints as well. She was so happy.

I have found positive results applying the concept of temporal macrocosms and microcosms many times, but Elizabeth's story is the one that has always stayed with me.

Each morning we have a window into our formative years; we have another opportunity to replace disordered patterns of our past with healthy ones, or reinforce positive ones that we have strived to create. Each new day ushers in a cascade of new possibilities and second chances.

While I haven't given it much thought, I doubt if there is a way to test this concept in a double-blind study. But I have seen it work beautifully to think outside the box, look for loopholes, and trust that together my patients and I can find healing possibilities.

32 Reflections on Part III

Really, my reflections on this part are similar to those in Part II. Practicing dexterity keeps our thinking flexible and our minds open and receptive to possibilities beyond our ability to predict. This can only further refine our confidence, humility, communication, empathy, and diagnostic accuracy, and result in better outcomes for our patients. In the final analysis, I think it would not be amiss to add dexterity to the list of qualities central to the art of medicine.

PART IV

Purity

Are We Medicine or Poison?

*Weapon, scripture, and water depend on their recipient
for consequent merits and demerits. So (a physician)
should purify his intellect for treatment of patients.*
CHARAKA[1]

*You need not dwell much on your personal character or
impurities of mind. It amounts to self pity. Although it is
a very happy augury to be conscious of one's shortcomings,
undue apprehension sometimes breeds morbidity...*
KIRPAL SINGH

*Friendliness and compassion towards the diseased,
attachment to the remediable, and emotional and mental
equilibrium with those who are moving towards the
end—this is the fourfold attitude of the physician.*
CHARAKA[2]

*... One worthy of being taught [medicine] should possess these
qualities: He should be calm, of noble nature, should not indulge in
mean acts, should have good looking eyes, mouth, and nasal ridge;
should have a thin, red, and clear tongue, with no abnormality
in teeth and lips. He should not speak with nasal utterance. He
should demonstrate restraint, should be humble, intelligent, endowed
with reasoning and memory, with broad mind, born in a family of*

physicians or having similar conduct, dedicated to truth, without deformity or impairment of senses, unpretentious, possess the ability to understand essence of the ideas, without anger and addictions; endowed with modesty, purity, good conduct, affection, dexterity, and sincerity, interested in study, devoted to understanding of ideas and practical knowledge without any distraction, having no greed or idleness. He should be compassionate to all creatures, follow all instructions of the teacher and should be attached to him.
CHARAKA[3]

The teacher should instruct the student of medicine, in their initial initiation, to live with celibacy, keeping beard and mustaches, speaking truth, not eating meat, using pure and intellect-promoting things without envy and possessing no weapons... The student should move without haughtiness, carefully, with concentrated mind, humbleness and constant vigilance, without jealousy... When you join the medical profession and wish success in work, prosperity, fame and heaven after death, you should always think of the welfare of all the living beings, keeping cow and brahmana before you. You should make efforts to provide health to patients by all means. You should not think ill of the patients even at the cost of your life. You should not approach the other's woman and any other's property, even in imagination. Your dress and accessories should be modest... You should not be addicted to drinking, indulge in sins or associated with sinners; you should speak smooth, pure, righteous, blissful, thankful, truthful, useful, and measured words.
CHARAKA[4]

A physician, having thoroughly studied the science of medicine, and fully pondered on and verified the truths he has assimilated, both by observation and practice, and having attained to that stage of lucid knowledge which would enable him to make a clear exposition of the science (whenever necessary), should open his medical practice with the permission of the king of his country. He should be clean in his habits and well shaved, and should not allow his nails to grow. He should wear white garments, put on a pair of shoes, carry a stick and an umbrella in his hands, and walk

about with a mild and benign look—as a friend of all created beings, ready to help all, and frank and friendly in his talk and demeanor, and never allowing the full control of his reason or intellectual powers to be in any way disturbed or interfered with.
SUSHRUTA[5]

Someone once asked my teacher what kind of medicine he preferred. He replied that he preferred the kind of medicine Jesus practiced, where someone is healed simply by touching the hem of Jesus's garment.

There are many stories, the world over, of miraculous cures taking place simply by being in the presence of a saintly person. These are profound examples of a human being becoming medicine. While not many may embody that degree of medical efficacy, it is not at all uncommon to feel either better or worse, to one degree or another, in anyone's presence. If the effect we have on others is good, we ourselves have become medicine—at least a little bit. If our effect on others is poor, we have become, to some extent, poisonous. This is not to say that we should conduct ourselves in such a way that we are constantly attempting to please others. It may be more the case that there are beneficial side effects to others as well as ourselves, when we ourselves are healthy—when we live in integrity, in such a way that our thoughts, hearts and tongues are in healthy alignment in our own beings. In cultivating such internal health, we practice not only the art of healthy living, but also the art of medicine.

33

Spiritual Powers vs. Effect of Character

The Ayurvedic classics, as well as Hippocrates himself,[1] stressed the importance of character in a physician. In Ayurveda, purity was expected of everyone. In a section devoted to how people should live in general, Charaka advised, "One should be devoted to celibacy, knowledge, charity, friendship, compassion, cheerfulness, patience, and calmness."[2] If this was mandated for everyone, it was even more important for physicians. Indeed, one would not be inducted into the study of medicine to begin with if their character were not impeccable, nor indeed even if the size, shape, and defining characteristics of their facial features fell outside certain parameters. Once inducted, the manner in which the student—and eventually the practitioner— dressed, talked, and even looked at people was scrutinized. The character of the physician had to be beyond reproach.

It may be more comfortable to emphasize techniques and data, and minimize the impact of our thoughts and behavior on our patients and their outcomes, but evidence suggests that this would be a mistake. Even clothes may have more of an impact than we often consider. Patients still overwhelmingly prefer their physicians in white coats.[3] Clothes may not make a man, but they do seem to make him appear more trustworthy. Whether or not we adopt dress codes, the character of a physician cannot be separated from her medical outcomes. As Dr. Cardona-Sanclemente says, "Because the Ayurvedic approach is through nature, one has to try to connect to one's own nature when practicing it."[4] When we purify our own nature and character, we bring that to the practice of medicine, and this has an effect. Modern studies show that patients' satisfaction with their doctors' approach, partnership, and communication skills—all reflective of their character—is a strong predictor of compliance and outcomes in both acute[5] and chronic[6] illnesses.

Once, in India, in a village called Manjhuvas, there lived a boy who was critically ill. His parents had taken him to many cities and doctors over the course of about a year, but he was now close to death. My guru went to see the boy, asked everybody else to leave the room, and gave the boy some of the very medicine the boy had already been taking. When my guru gave the boy this medicine with his own hands, the boy immediately improved. It took about 20 days for the boy to fully regain his strength, but the turning point was when he received the medicine from my guru's hands.[7]

My guru said that there was no miracle in this, and it was not due to his spiritual powers that the child had been cured. It was simply a side effect we see when a practitioner leads a pure life and has disciplined thoughts. Just as the environment in which we treat a patient can serve to support his health, so too can our own character. In fact, our intent to heal is not even necessary. The healing happens as a side effect. We may all be able to think of a time when we felt healed by being in someone's presence even if they weren't aware of ours—perhaps listening to a speaker or singer or watching a performance or performer. When there is intent, though, perhaps there is even more effect.

There is a saying in India that even if a holy man gives a little bit of ash as medicine, it will work and, indeed, stories like this abound. Sometimes it is with ash. Sometimes with water. Sometimes it is with other simple remedies that result in profound effects.

My guru tells a story of a *vaidya* in his village who had amazing results with three very simple remedies. He always prescribed only one of three remedies. I think one was a gourd. Not positive about that. I don't remember what the other two were. That's not the point of the story. The point is that the *vaidya* had wonderful success with his three simple remedies, and patients would come from far and wide to be treated by him. His own son then went to and graduated from a six-year government Ayurveda college, and when his father passed away, he went into practice, with a large pharmacy. After some time, he went to my guru and asked why he wasn't having as much success as his father. After all, he prescribed many formulas and remedies, while his father had only three simple medicines. My guru told him that it was because his father had lived a very pure life and had disciplined his mind.

The ability to accurately identify and comprehend the mental conditions of other people is repeatedly shown to be an important factor in developing and experiencing empathy, and it has been demonstrated that meditation practices that cultivate compassion enhance empathic accuracy.[8] When we cultivate our character, through meditative and reflective practices, our senses become less polluted, so we are able to more clearly perceive the reality of and the Good in our patients. Clearer perception leads to greater empathy. Greater empathy leads to improved outcomes.

My guru, a *vaidya* himself, said that the original Ayurvedic preceptors taught their students:

> It is very important for you to have good character, because only then will the healing you are doing be beneficial to the patient. If your character is not good, your treatment will not give any benefit to your patient. But if you have good character, if you are chaste, then it can have a direct effect on the patient, and even if you only give him a little medicine, he can become all right.[9]

In fact, when all else fails—if we feel we do not know anything, if we have little experience and very little education in other sciences that could add to our ability to practice dexterous medicine—still there is hope if we can strive towards purity. We can do this in many ways, including efforts at purifying and disciplining the senses, as we saw in Chapter 2 earlier.

My guru said that even if a doctor doesn't have sophisticated knowledge of pathology and medicine, if she possesses good character, then her character would come to her aid.[10] He said:

> If you are pure, and with your pure hands you give anything to anyone, it will carry the best effect, and that person will definitely get healed…if there is any doctor who has a chaste life, who is doing even a little bit of meditation, no matter what medicine he gives to the patients, they will be healed. Besides the medicine, the doctor's own charging will also work to remove the sicknesses. If there is any complicated sickness, it may take

time, but if the doctor has a good life, if he is chaste and if he has good thoughts, all these will have an effect on the patient also.[11]

Again, this does not mean someone is healing through their spiritual power. It is nothing that lofty, tricky, or questionable. It is simply a side effect of the practitioner's integrity and purity.

Because a doctor's belief, as we have seen in Chapter 17, "Confidence vs. Cockiness," plays a significant role in a patient's outcome, and because the patient's level of optimism versus pessimism also affects their outcome, as we have seen in Chapter 19, our patients should leave our offices feeling more hopeful. In other words, if the same patient with the same disorder sees two different doctors, it is most beneficial for that patient to choose the one that makes her feel the most hopeful and positive, because it is with this doctor that she is more likely to have a positive outcome. As a couple of long-time TCM practitioners write, "The patient needs to feel that she has a will and a purpose in life when she leaves your office. This is not only a part of the diagnosis, it is part of the treatment..."[12] One man's meat is another man's poison: a relationship and approach that will work well for one patient may be detrimental to another. One way or another, for each patient, a particular doctor can act as a poison or as medicine.

34

The Mechanics of Emotional Contagion

Who Affects Whom?

You're always treating yourself.
ANONYMOUS

Who Affects Whom?

One of the most common questions I am asked about private practice is some variation of, "How do you keep from feeling depleted or taking on your patients' emotions or difficulties?" There are no doubt a number of answers to this, but here are a few observations.

The first is simple. Working with patients is an activity that uses certain mental, emotional, and possibly physical (depending on your modality) muscles that we may not necessarily use outside our practice. Like any muscles, they require repetition and time to become strong.

When we are first in practice, we may feel more easily fatigued, as a rule, than we do later on. As we gain more experience, we may still have the odd day when we feel easily fatigued. This may not be due to patients' emotions or even our own. It may just be due to our biorhythms or having a low-energy day for whatever reason. Or maybe we are simply working too much, outspending our own emotional, mental, physical, or spiritual resources. In which case, we might need to work less.

This happened to me. To practice what is in this book takes time, presence of mind, and being healthy myself. At a certain point, my teaching, writing, and traveling were picking up, and I had to make choices about where to put my energy. I was teaching the importance of not overextending ourselves and the very important role stress plays in health. It would have been hypocritical to keep trying to do it all. So, some years ago, I first cut my practice to part time and then, as my teaching and writing responsibilities increased further, I closed my practice. Sometimes we are just working too much.

If we are not working too much, our muscles are strong, and we are sturdy—this may suffice for most days and situations, but occasionally it may not be enough. There may be certain emotions, situations, or behaviors of a particular patient that find their way under our skin and knock us off center. This can be humbling. We can go along for days, months, years feeling centered, and then a particular patient, in one brief interaction or phone message, can shake us to the core. For whatever reason. Somehow a particular behavior, emotion, or situation is strong enough to impact a place in us that feels weak, shaky or vulnerable.

Here it is useful to ask, "Who affects whom?"

There is (yet another) story from India. A well-behaved boy takes up company with a mischievous boy. The father of the well-behaved boy sits him down and tells him he does not want him to associate with the other boy, as he will be a bad influence. The child replies, "Father, I can play with him without becoming mischievous myself." The father responds by asking the child to bring him a piece of coal with his bare hands, but be sure not to blacken them. The son observes, "That is impossible. How can I touch the coal without getting blackened?" In the same way, his father says, how can he expect to play with the other boy without being affected?

The same question could be asked by the father of the mischievous boy. This father may wish his son to associate with a boy of fine character, hoping the boy's good behavior will rub off on his son.

So, who affects whom? Do we heal patients, or do they somehow contaminate us? While I am aware that this may sound judgmental or nasty, it is not an uncommon perspective or question. Do we affect our patients, or do they affect us? Do we all influence each other with our behavior and experience? While it may certainly be the case that we affect each other, it is worth looking at how this dynamic might work.

Mirror Neurons and Empathy

One way of understanding how we affect each other is to understand the implications associated with the fact that we all possess mirror neurons. A mirror neuron is a nerve cell that fires when we act *and* when we see someone else act.

For example, if I pick up a glass, certain motor neurons will fire in my brain. But even if I simply *watch* someone else pick up a glass, about 20 percent of those neurons will still fire. The same applies to being touched and watching someone else be touched. If I watch Alice being caressed, it activates a subset of the same neurons in my brain as if I were being caressed in the same way. This is why people with phantom limb pain can feel relief just watching someone else's limb get massaged. It is one reason why we feel joy at another's joy, sorrow for another's sorrow, why people laugh when they watch movies of babies laughing, or—in a different vein but equally powerful application—feel aroused watching porn.

As neuroscientist V. S. Ramachandran says, "It is as though this neuron was adopting the other person's point of view."[1] Indeed, scientists speculate that this is partially how human beings learn empathy. (We looked at this a little in Chapter 2, in the section on refining our ability to feel or touch.) Part of us literally experiences what we see another person experience, to one degree or another. What is happening to them is also happening to us, only on a smaller scale.

Since a subset of my own neurons fire when I watch somebody else being caressed, why don't I believe that I myself am being caressed? First of all, perhaps because it is a smaller percentage of the neurons firing than if I were actually being caressed, but also because the touch receptors on my skin are sending messages to my brain that let me know I am not being touched. That's the difference between empathy and first-hand experience. Science has shown, in fact, that if someone's arm has gone to sleep, he *will* feel the sensation of being touched on the arm if he sees someone else's arm being touched. *If it weren't for our skin and our sense of touch, we could not discern the difference between experience and empathy.*[2]

Mirror neurons represent both good news and bad news for the doctor–patient relationship. The good news is that if we are centered, calm, present, and kind, our patients will feel somewhat the same way in their bodies. The bad news? If our patients are anxiety-ridden, suspicious, in pain, or in an otherwise uncomfortable state of being, we experience their experience, albeit to a lesser degree. Perhaps this is one reason why some practitioners report feeling drained at the end of a day of treating patients.

Do we affect our patients, or do they affect us? The answer is probably yes. If we spend time with our patients and they are troubled, how do we remain unaffected? If patients' verbal or non-verbal communication—their thoughts, emotions, or words—are troubled, how do we avoid feeling troubled ourselves?

Establishing a Strong Pattern: He with the Deepest Breath Wins

> *When both patient and practitioner are in communication with their own spirits, the communication with Heaven is open.*
> CLAUDE LARRE AND ELISABETH ROCHAT DE LA VALLEE[3]

Many years ago I read a passage in an old Indian text. It was something archaic like, "He with the deepest breath wins." (I am taking liberties with this.) At the time I read it, it struck me, but I didn't fully appreciate the meaning—or at least the meaning I eventually gleaned from it—until later.

Because of the intimate connection between breath and *prana* in the classics, I have come to think that one of the possible meanings of that passage relates to *prana* as much or more than to breath. In Ayurveda or TCM, we might say that *prana* or *qi* moves in certain patterns in a person. So one way to understand that passage is: the stronger and more ingrained the *pranic* pattern is in a person, the more likely it is to affect others, rather than be affected by others. Let us look at a few examples.

Once there was a group of disciples milling around the courtyard of my teacher's ashram. Suddenly there entered a *sadhu* who was absolutely enraged—so enraged, in fact, that my friend, who was present at the time, said the *sadhu* was literally frothing at the mouth. All the disciples became paralyzed with shock by what they were seeing. Nobody knew what to do as the *sadhu* continued to froth and fume. Then our teacher walked into the courtyard, placed his hands on the man's head, and then ran his hands down the *sadhu's* body, as if draining the rage out of his body and into the ground. The *sadhu's* body and mind became meek and sweet, and he became like putty in the guru's hands.

What was happening here? Who can say? But one way to understand it is that the *sadhu's* pattern of *prana* and behavior—his alignment with his intense emotion—was stronger than the default pattern going on in all the disciples, thus imbuing the atmosphere with his rage and paralyzing them all. But the teacher's pattern of *prana* and behavior—his alignment with something greater that kept him steady and calm—was even stronger than the *sadhu's*, so he was able to establish a new dominant pattern.

An admittedly more banal (and rehearsed) example comes to mind. I once saw Cher in concert. There were dozens of very talented performers, dancers, and acrobats on stage, but when Cher walked on, it didn't matter how amazing the others were. Cher commanded total attention and suffused the moment with Cher energy. Completely.

There is Western scientific evidence that biological changes occur when we are in the proximity of someone with a strong emotion or condition. Consider the results of a study on the biological changes in members of a wedding party. Perhaps predictably, the bride measured highest for levels of oxytocin, a hormone released when people feel connected and loving. More surprising was that oxytocin levels were also higher than normal in people hanging around the bride.[4] The bride had the dominant biological pattern, and that affected the emotional and physiological patterns of everyone in contact with her. They didn't have to speak with her. They didn't have to touch her. She didn't have to touch them. People's thoughts and emotions, and therefore their biology, changed just by focusing on the radiant bride and being in her proximity.

In each of these examples—the *sadhu*, Cher, and the bride—people were paying attention to and being influenced by the dominant expression and experience of another person. This may happen whenever two or more people are together, to greater or lesser degrees. Consider how it feels to walk into a tense room versus a room that is almost palpably emanating love? Think of entering a courtroom versus making a visit to Amma ji, the hugging woman saint.

Thoughts and emotions create biology and particular *pranic* patterns. When we do something that commands the attention of others, their subsequent thoughts, emotions, and experiences create their biological and *pranic* patterns. In other words, the one with the deepest *pranic* pattern wins.

If we consider this in light of the mirror neuron phenomenon, we see that, at least to a small degree, we become each other when we focus on each other. This might be one of the reasons that a doctor can *be* medicine. The doctor is not the only party experiencing empathy—or becoming the other. It works both ways. The patient experiences empathy too. When we pay attention to the patient, we experience what they experience, at least to a small degree. If we are also paying attention to our internal environment at that moment, we can choose to compassionately address and heal what we experience within. Meanwhile, our patient, by simply paying attention to us, experiences what we experience, at least to a small degree. So, if we have healed the problem, even to a small extent, in ourselves, the patient will be rearranged accordingly and experience at least a small measure of healing.

How do I heal myself, moment to moment? I can always work towards creating a harmonious internal environment, through internal awareness and continuous remembrance to keep my own *prana* smooth and flowing. So, as a physician, I am continuously treating myself and a side effect of this is that the patient can experience relief as well.

There are many, many ways in which human beings affect each other: the language we use, the clothes we wear, our character, actions, words, and thoughts. If we work diligently to reinforce healthy patterns in our life, we may create strong ones.

My guru told me a physician's thoughts should be very pure, he should be very intelligent, he should not himself have sick thoughts, and he should regularly engage in his spiritual practices. Habitual dedication to building, maintaining, and improving our physical, emotional, and spiritual health is imperative in supporting a pattern strong enough to stand up to the onslaught of the myriad energies we encounter in a busy medical practice. Or in life in general. Doing so transforms us and, therefore, helps our patients.

When we are in integrity, we are authentically, wholly ourselves, without trying to please, hide, show off, fix or manipulate a situation. We surrender to, and accept, reality. This requires intention and practice, but the pay-off is worth it. This state of being is a refuge for authenticity. It gives our patients permission to accept reality too, and to situate in their own authenticity and wholeness, and meaning descends to bless us both.

Does this mean that our pure state of mind is dominating our patient's soiled mind? Not so. What I think it means is that rather than relying on the strength of our own individual pattern, we are relying on something that is stronger than either of us, and that has the strength to sustain us both. When we become situated in that strength, it overwhelms the inauthentic, petty, disturbed goings-on in the minds and hearts of us both.

Once, some disciples were in the Himalayas with my teacher. One of them mused, "Wouldn't it be wonderful for Master to give us strength enough to climb that mountain!" My teacher responded, "Better to request God to drag you up the mountain."

If we daily practice aligning with and trusting the Good Orderly Direction (G.O.D.) of life and nature—Something Bigger Than Ourselves—we are relying on a very strong pattern. In so doing, we invite our patients to join the party—to align as well with a source of strength so many have found in dire circumstances, rather than lean on our personal strength, wisdom, or experience. This supports a partnership instead of a dynamic that implies that the physician is a savior.

So rather than relying on our own strong pattern or risking being emotionally rearranged by the strong patterns of our patients, if we align with something truly strong, our patients experience our stability and confidence, and it can have an immediate therapeutic effect, especially as we are about to explore, when we employ love and focus. Then it is not so much a question of who wins, but a way to facilitate harmony with anyone at any time.

35

Supporting Change Through Appropriate Familiarity, Love, and Focus

So many of us—our patients and ourselves—are looking for change. We want to replace unhealthy habits and patterns with healthy ones. The problem is old patterns can be stubborn and new ones can seem, well, boring. We often find it a bit of a forced march to engage in healthy practices. We can even feel cool and rebellious when resisting these practices. So can patients.

We have already looked at how aligning ourselves with Something Truly Strong can have a therapeutic effect on others. We can also consciously support another's receptivity to change by fostering appropriate familiarity, and employing love and focus. Each plays a unique role in healing.

Let us look first at the role of familiarity. In Part I we looked at our ability to increase our own empathic abilities. How we behave can also invite empathy in others—a factor that increases their receptivity to change. In a McGill University study published in the journal *Current Biology* in January 2015, researchers found emotional contagion—a component of empathy—to work much more effectively when people feel familiar with each other than when they were strangers.[1] It also didn't take a lot to turn strangers into friends and, as lead researcher Professor Jeff Mogil said, "generate meaningful levels of empathy."[2] Simply playing a few Beatles songs together on the video game Rock Band® was sufficient. It took about 15 minutes. Consider how bonded children feel at summer camp after just a few games, or sports fans of the same team. This may be rather beneficial for doctor–patient relationships as well—to feel we are on the same team.

We have a greater ability to affect each other when we feel connected. And it may not take a lot to achieve that connectivity. We can look for common ground and shared experience with almost anybody the first time we sit with them and review their health history together. If we are too busy to do this, we may maintain "stranger" status, a relationship wherein empathy doesn't flow well. It is well worth that 15 minutes at our first meeting, to establish a relationship that fosters change.

Once bonded in appropriate familiarity, love and focus can do the rest.

When we experience stubborn patterns of behavior, thinking, or illness that despite a great deal of effort won't budge, it can feel like these patterns are etched in cement. They are so intractable, so long-standing, and so entrenched in our bodies and personalities, they might as well be.

Wouldn't it be nice if there were a magic serum that would soften that cement to allow change? There is. It is called oxytocin.

Oxytocin makes the brain—and therefore us—more malleable and receptive to new impressions and pathways. Sometimes called the love hormone or the cuddle hormone, it increases when we love and feel loved.

If we provide a safe, loving environment for our patients, both their and our oxytocin levels can increase and smooth the way for change.

Once we have softened the cement, we need an etching tool to create a new pathway. There is such a tool. It is called focus.

When we are infants and young children developing into who we will become, there is a part of the brain called the nucleus basalis, which is constantly active. The nucleus basalis is related to the creation of new neural pathways. When it is on, pathways are created easily. This is why we describe children as sponges. They soak up new languages and skills more quickly than adults because of their receptivity to new impressions, thanks to the nucleus basalis.

However, keeping so many neural pathways alive and active requires a tremendous amount of energy—apparently an unsustainable amount because, around puberty, the nucleus basalis turns off. Our brains preserve active patterns and pathways, but prune away dormant or rarely used ones. This conserves energy, but also makes it more difficult to create new patterns and pathways.

So how do we do this after puberty?

Happily, when we wish to form a new pathway, there is a simple way to reactivate the nucleus basalis. Focus. Concentration is one of the few "on" switches to reactivate the nucleus basalis, allowing us once again to create new neural pathways efficiently.

In summary, when we foster appropriate familiarity, our relationship with a patient can move quickly from reserved to friendly—territory more conducive to transformation. Then the combination of love, which stimulates oxytocin and makes us even more receptive to change, and concentrated focus, which allows us to more readily create new patterns, becomes a powerful blend that brings real change within the realm of possibility.

When we provide a loving environment for our patients, and when we consider together how and what to focus on to help shift old patterns, patients' oxytocin levels may rise. They can receive inspiration for focus, and change may be more easily within their grasp.

36 Good Company

The doctor should discourse with other doctors to promote
pursuit and advancement of knowledge, dexterity, etc.
CHARAKA[1]

When I was barely eight years old, my guru sent me a letter in which he wrote, "Keep good company. Good company makes a man great." If we consult with patients all day and find ourselves tiring in spirit, we may need to feed our sense of love, hope, and goodness in other ways. If we meet with other physicians or kindred spirits committed to similar goals and ideals, we will more likely be able to maintain healthy patterns, perspectives, and alignment with Something Greater Than Ourselves.

Our own mental, emotional, physical, and spiritual hygiene is up to us. To keep it in order, it helps to consistently choose to be aware of our limitations, strengths, aspirations, and practices, and choose to support the good stuff while weeding out the other stuff.

What is good company? I have considered this a lot. I have come to think that good company is anyone who has a good effect on me. This can also be a function, though, of what I choose to focus on in them. We've seen that *prana* follows that upon which we are focused. We feed what we focus on.

Charaka tells us that for the wise, the whole world is a teacher, and we should learn "excellence of conduct" even from those we may consider to be enemies.[2] Recently I finished watched an entire season of a program that starred a couple of morally repugnant characters. Though I was sufficiently disgusted to stop watching the show after a few episodes, I was sufficiently fascinated that I returned to it after some time, and finished the season. I admitted this to a friend who asked what I had gotten out of it. Upon reflection, I realized that though the characters had made choices I disagreed with, I admired their fortitude and backbone. They didn't care what people thought of them. When situations looked bleak, they adjusted. Granted, I wouldn't call these characters "good company" or seek out such company (and I expect that if I spent much time with or watching people like this it could have a poor effect on me), but if I focus on what I admire in them—or anybody—that may be what I feed in myself. Maybe, just maybe, I can play with the charcoal without blackening my hands...too badly.

Ultimately, we can pay close attention to whether something or someone is having a good effect on us or not. In general, if we choose to adopt and focus on qualities in others that support a healthy mind and body, and learn from any qualities that seem obstructive, we may be able to nourish character rather than erode it.

If we remain vigilant about how the influences in our environment, thoughts, diet, and life affect us, we may better understand and assimilate them, and empathize with the way our patients are affected as well. All these elements create the context of our lives. It may be that all the dietary changes and herbal remedies we adopt are not sufficient to address our maladies if the company we keep is not "good company."

37 Physical Purification

There is a rather famous story (though the particulars differ a bit in different versions): once a woman took a long journey to bring her son to Mahatma Gandhi, and requested Gandhi ji to tell her son to stop eating sugar. Gandhi ji asked the woman to return in a week. When the woman returned with her son the following week, Gandhi ji told her son to stop eating sugar. The woman is said to have asked Gandhi ji why he couldn't have just told her son this when they came the first time. Gandhi ji reportedly smiled and said, "I was not qualified to advise the boy. At that time, I, too, was eating lots of sugar."

Once, many years ago, some years after quitting smoking, I was sneaking a cigarette with a friend in an alley behind (*drum roll*) The Ayurvedic Institute, where I worked and studied at the time. The founder of the Institute, my boss, friend, and world-renowned Ayurvedic physician Dr. Vasant Lad, drove by and saw us. He didn't say anything. Months later, in a clinical setting, he told the students present, including me, something that touched my heart. I forget his exact words, but I remember their gentle, sweet tone and their gist: we cannot expect our patients to do that which we ourselves cannot do.

This is rather self-evident, but it bears aiming for to the best of our abilities. I once heard from a traditionally trained practitioner of TCM that he was taught not to trust practitioners who don't fast on some regular basis. If we don't practice the discipline necessary to maintain our own health, at least on some regular basis, what kind of effect will our words carry when we counsel patients on their health?

I have learned, through various traditions, that there is very little power in empty words, whereas our personal experience enlivens them, rendering them potent.

Jeanette arrived for her first consultation. Sometime during the intake she said, somewhat sheepishly, that she had been told by an old, experienced Chinese medical doctor that one should not trust TCM practitioners who do not have moxa scars on both Stomach 36 points—a point near each knee. (There is a tradition, though rarely employed in Western countries, whereby moxa—a herb—is burned on these points to increase stamina, *qi*, and blood. Doing this leaves scars.) She was delighted when I rolled up my pants legs and revealed two dime-sized scars.

Not everyone has to fast or burn their legs. There is no specific rite-of-passage to which we must all submit in order to be effective physicians. And we don't have to have perfect health. I have studied with, and enjoyed the company of, many incredible, effective, brilliant physicians. I have never met one who enjoys both perfect physical and mental health.

It doesn't do to wallow in self-loathing or reproach if we miss the mark—if we fall short of purity sometimes, many times, or—it could be argued—anytime.

We don't have to be perfect (thank heavens) but, in the same way that we may know little but we and our patients benefit from our pursuit of knowledge, though we may not be pure, there are benefits to the pursuit of purification.

Shamans, healers, and doctors from many traditions have known the value of purification in healing and tried to purify themselves physically as well as mentally, through sweat lodges and spiritual retreats. Purifying themselves helps them perceive their patients more clearly.

Pursuing physical health and purification through such practices, and even through adhering to healthy dietary and lifestyle practices ourselves, supports mental and sensory health and purification, as we generally need to discipline our senses in order to comply with dietary and health regimens. When we are acquainted with discipline, we may have more empathy for what our patients are going through, and our words may carry greater weight and inspiration. My teacher used to say we can be inspired because, "What man has done, man can do."

38 Reflections on Part IV

In Part I, we looked at the pursuit of theoretical knowledge. In Part II, we looked at putting the theory we've learned into practice with our patients. In Part III, we explored thinking outside the box. In this fourth part, we prioritize putting the theory we've learned into practice with our own physical health and personal character, and explore the effects that may have on patients. And, lo, the effects are good.

When we purify ourselves, we align with a force of Good. If we do this consistently and sincerely, it becomes a strong habit and experience, and it may serve as an invitation or permission for patients to do the same. When we align with Good, we focus on it. When we focus on it, we feed it. When we feed it—either in our patients or ourselves—we strengthen it. They and we become it, at least to some extent. When we are aligned with Good and our patients focus on us, Good is further reinforced, at least to some extent. So no matter the ultimate outcome, when we align with Good, part of the effect is that the Good is strengthened in both physician and patient. To the extent that Good is strengthened in the physician is the extent to which she has become medicine.

PART V

The Four Qualities of Effective Medicine

Abundance, suitability, multiple forms and
potency—these are the four qualities of drugs.
CHARAKA[1]

If you remember from the Introduction to this book, Charaka lists four components of successful treatment: the physician, the nurse, the medicine, and the patient. Because the physician is directly responsible for the medicine component, it is useful here to consider the art of prescription in the context of the art of medicine.

In Brazil, in the summer of 2010, I had the good fortune to meet and enjoy the company of Dona Francisca, a shaman and medicine woman from the Yawanawa (pronounced "shawah nawah") tribe, a two-day boat ride up the Amazon. Mother to 11 of her own children, Dona Francisca had delivered between one and two thousand babies, her first when she was 15 years old. She had apprenticed as a medicine woman since she was five or six years old.

Among other things, Dona Francisca talked about how we treat our medicinal plants. She said that, like humans, plants feel pain, and just as we would not appreciate someone pulling, scratching, or grabbing us, plants also shrink against rough, thoughtless treatment. She said that when we harvest plants in a violent, careless manner, without asking their permission or praying, they may cause disease in our patients, in us, and for the planet.

With the increasing popularity of CAM and the herbal remedies on which it relies, how we grow, gather, and prescribe plant medicine may be more important now than ever before. But in our hunger for new remedies and knowledge, and due to the demands of a private practice and busy lives, it can be easy to overlook this.

Many indigenous medical traditions pay close attention to the relationship between doctor and medicine. The Ayurvedic classics are no exception, and they provide detailed instructions about herbal collection methods. For example, along with instructions on the appropriate time and season for collection, Charaka says:

> One should collect the various parts of these plants while facing towards the east or north after performing auspicious rites in a spirit of compassion, while living a pure life, while wearing white dress, after offering prayers to the gods, Asvins, cows, and Brahmins, and while observing fast.
>
> The collected plant products should be kept in appropriate containers well covered with a lid, and hung on a swing. The storeroom should have doors facing towards the east or the north... Flower offerings and sacrificial rituals should be performed in the storeroom every day...[2]

According to Charaka, then, it is important to practice what we learned in Part IV before interacting with plants.

While it is common practice in many medical traditions for the physician to choose the medicine for her patients, in many indigenous forms of medicine, it works in reverse. In these, the shaman or practitioner establishes a respectful rapport with the plant medicine, and then the plants let the shaman or practitioner know when they will be a good fit for a patient.

Charaka was aware that it was not always practical or possible for physicians to personally know and oversee how medicines are identified, grown, harvested, stored, distributed, prescribed, and consumed. And perhaps he was aware that it was not in the nature of every physician to be interested in this work. He did suggest that someone should be, though, and that goatherds, shepherds, cowherds, and other forest dwellers could do much of the work.[3]

In the modern world, our herbs can be grown in a sustainable and respectful manner, harvested or collected by gardeners, and the whole process overseen by conscientious companies that take it upon themselves to follow the spirit of the texts as much as possible. And it is possible for physicians to carefully choose from which companies they purchase their herbs. As consumers of groceries vote with their forks and dollars, so do physicians affect plants, patients, and the planet by where they purchase their medicines.

Just as there are four qualities that are important to be a good physician, there are four qualities Charaka lists that are important for medicine to be effective: abundance, suitability, multiple forms, and potency.[4]

Each of these qualities is related to the others, and to our relationship with plants.

39 Abundance

In 2002, *The Hindu* reported that there were 143 Ayurvedic plants that were on restricted lists for trade and export, including 114 plant species submitted by wildlife authorities and 29 by India's Commerce Ministry.[1] As demand exceeds supply, the plant medicine on which we rely is becoming less and less abundant. Indeed, we have already seen precious plants and strong medicinal plants like kutki, jatamamsi, and sandalwood harvested to the point of endangerment.

In 2010, a *vaidya* in South India told me that when doctors are unable to use a plant because of its restricted status, they find substitute herbs. While this approach may conform to Charaka's dictum to the letter, it may be prudent to consider what will happen when the substitute herbs, too, become over-harvested.

Using substitute herbs is not a long-term solution. If we over-harvest one, use it up, and then over-harvest another, we simply strain two species instead of one.

In Jared Diamond's book, *Collapse: How Societies Choose to Fail or Succeed*, Diamond relates how certain cultures and communities became extinct over the millennia. Each time, extinction followed exploitation of natural resources without replenishing them. Eventually the last tree was chopped down, the last source of water polluted, and the last crucial resource harvested until there was nothing left. The people perished along with their resources.

It would certainly be prudent to grow herbs in a sustainable way, but there are more direct ways to protect plant medicine.

The reasons abundance is threatened may well relate to the other three qualities that efficacious medicine must possess: suitability, multiple form, and potency.

40 Suitability

Consideration of whether a particular plant medicine is suitable for a particular patient is a human-centric perspective. This is understandable, but we might also consider whether it is suitable for the plant.

How do we know if a specific plant is suitable medicine for a patient? For the shaman, who has a relationship with her local plants, the plants themselves may suggest their suitability for a particular patient. Otherwise, suitability may be related to the quality of abundance. If our plants are over-harvested to the point of making the restricted and endangered lists, perhaps they are unsuitable for use as medicine.

It is not uncommon today to overuse or misuse nature's bounty by overeating in general, or consuming food and drinks that have been adulterated or contaminated with pesticides and insecticides, or that are so highly processed they are more likely to create disease. When all this makes us sick, we return to nature's cupboards to consume more plants, in the form of medicine. It may serve equally well—or better—to simply stop the practices that led to the problems in the first place. In these cases, perhaps the more suitable medicine would be to offer lifestyle and diet counseling first, before prescribing herbs and supplements.

If we still consider herbal medicine to be necessary, we might consider whether a patient is likely to follow through with taking the herbs we prescribe.[1] If not, it may be more prudent, again, to offer lifestyle and dietary recommendations, and save the plants for the patients who will actually take them. Many patients find the taste of herbs so unpleasant that they stop taking them. Far too often, we take a dose or two, and put the rest in the back of a cabinet. This wasted plant might otherwise have been used to ease another's suffering, or been left to grow and contribute to its ecosystem.

Charaka tells us that there is nothing in the world that is not therapeutic in appropriate conditions and situations.[2] If this is the case, we should be able to easily find something that is abundant, suits the patient's sensibilities, pocketbook, and constitution, and will not strain the coffers of the earth's resources. This will suit the plants as well as our patients.

In the ancient herbal compendium *Dravyagunavignyana,* a commentary says that the sage physician Vagbhata[3] was inclined to use single herb remedies: he recommended the use of a single herb or remedy in 42 of 55 cases.[4] While certain cases may require formulations of multiple herbs, we should not overlook the possibility that a single herb—if known, cultivated, harvested, and prescribed with love and respect—could be potent medicine. Why use multiple plants when one is sufficient? Indeed, why use one, when lifestyle and dietary changes will suffice?

41 Multiple Form

Determining the number of plant species on earth right now is not very easy. As of 2014, The Plant List, an authoritative working list of all known plant species, listed 350,699 accepted plant species.[1]

Of these hundreds of thousands of plant species, ecologist and professor Tom Lovejoy, who has worked in the Brazilian Amazon since 1965, informs us that there is not even one species we can claim to understand.[2] Whether or not we fully understand any species, we do know something of some of them, and we benefit greatly for our knowledge. As of the year 2000, only about 120 distinct chemical substances considered important drugs were derived from plants.[3] The medical potential of plants has only begun to be tapped, but we may never have the opportunity to realize that potential.

It has been estimated that by the year 2000, some 10 percent of the species of plants on our earth had already become extinct.[4] A hundred years ago, the human population stood at about one billion. Now we are well over six billion. The rate at which we are consuming our natural resources is increasing exponentially.

- While obtaining exact figures seems impossible, experts agree that we lose more than 80,000 acres—and degrade 80,000 more—of tropical rainforest every day. With this devastation, we lose about 135 animal, insect, and plant species every day. *That is nearly 50,000 species per year.* Since rainforests are home to about 50 percent of the world's species, and a quarter of our modern pharmaceuticals are derived from ingredients acquired there, rainforests are our living pharmacy. And considering that less than 1 percent of rainforest trees and plants have been tested for curative properties, it is also a largely untapped pharmacy.[5]

Along with the drastic reduction in plant diversity—that is, "multiple forms," as Charaka called it—the guardians and stewards who have intimate and vast knowledge of plants are also disappearing. In 1993, Harvard professor and explorer of the Amazon, Richard Evans Schultes, wrote that over 90 Brazilian tribes had become extinct since the turn of the 20th century.[6] As a planet, we have already suffered incalculable loss.

If we try to address the abundance problem by growing huge crops of single herbs, we automatically ignore the importance of diversity. Though we currently live in a world that favors monoculture over diversity, it is a short-sighted preference, and has rarely been nature's preference. Single-species crops generally require heavy use of toxic chemicals, insecticides, fungicides, and pesticides. And even if we can figure out how to grow single-species crops without the uses of toxins, whenever we change the environment in which a plant grows, we also change how it grows.

Consider *Impatiens pallida* (yellow jewelweed).[7] When these plants grow next to unrelated plants, they work hard to compete for resources. They grow bigger leaves to better crowd out other species and capture more sunlight, and they spread their root systems wider to more effectively capture nutrients. They become the strongest plants they can be. When they grow strong, it forces other species in the ecosystem to find their own niches, wherein they too can flourish. In order to survive, each species is forced to compete, become strong, unique, and more potent.

In the absence of diversity, *Impatiens* behave very differently. When they grow alongside their relatives, they sacrifice some of their individual vitality, growing smaller leaves and meeker root systems for the good of their kin. Diversity forces them to become stronger. Being surrounded by their kin breeds mediocrity.

This is worth considering when we attempt to grow medicinal (or other) plants that have historically been wild-crafted in diverse habitats outside their native habitat or in mono crops. A herb grown in a diverse plant community or native habitat could be more potent than one in a contrived habitat or monoculture. At the very least, it is likely that by growing medicinal plants in such a way, we are altering their qualities and therefore the effects they will have on us.

42 Potency

*It is not that the various drugs and diets act only by virtue of
their qualities. In fact, they act by virtue of their own nature or
qualities— or both— on a proper occasion, in a given location,
in appropriate conditions and situation. The effect so produced is
considered to be their action (karma); the factor responsible for the
manifestation of the effect is known as virya; where they act is the
adhisthana; When they act is the time. How they act is the upaya
or mode of action. What they accomplish is the achievement.*
CHARAKA[1]

*O! Agnivesa, some abnormalities are now appearing in the
stars, planets, moon, sun, air, fire and directions. This forecasts
abnormality in the coming seasons. Very soon, the earth will cease
to manifest proper tastes, potency, vipaka and specific actions in
drugs. This is bound to result in the widespread manifestation
of diseases. Therefore, O Agnivesa, all of you should collect
drugs before the time of destruction and before the earth loses
its fertility leading to the impairment of the taste, potency,
vipaka and specific action of drugs grown over it. We shall
administer these drugs having correct taste, potency, vipaka and
specific action to such of our patients as are dependent upon us
and whom we desire to treat (because of the curability of their
ailments). It is not difficult to treat epidemic diseases, provided
the drugs are collected, preserved and administered properly.*
CHARAKA[2]

Of the four qualities necessary for effective medicine, potency may be the most intriguing. How humans grow and treat plants affects the plants' qualities and behavior. These qualities and behavior, in turn, determine plants' potency and effects on humans.

That plants respond to stimuli is not breaking news. In the early 1900s, Dr. Jagadis Chandra Bose (1858–1937) demonstrated that plants feel pain and respond to human intent much as animals do, and their growth is enhanced or thwarted by exposure to sweet music or loud, harsh sounds, respectively.[3]

In the 1960s, inspired by Bose's work, former CIA interrogation specialist Cleve Backster strove to learn more about the extent to which plants were aware of and affected by their environments. He attached polygraph sensors to plants, and found that they responded to harmful thoughts as well as actions. They were aware of each other and reacted to the deaths of fellow plants, and even other species. They were affected by non-local events, as well as those in their immediate environment, reacting instantaneously to events occurring thousands of miles away. They could also anticipate both positive and negative events.[4]

While Backster's work might seem far-fetched, or an extreme example of anthropomorphosis, it is widely studied and accepted as fact that plants regularly sense, communicate with, and react to their environment in various ways, including changing their chemistry and behavior.[5]

How do plants sense their environments? While they don't have nervous systems or obvious sense organs as animals do, they have evolved highly sophisticated and dynamically responsive versions of them in their network of chloroplasts, stromules, photoelectrophysiological signaling (PEPS) circuits, bundle sheath cells, and cellular light memory.[6]

Because plants are unable to escape from environmental stresses, they have evolved intricate biological responses. There are many fascinating examples of this. For example, when plants "hear" insect herbivores munching on a leaf, the plants react by secreting defensive chemicals.[7]

Consider, too, the foliage of the "sensitive plant" (*Mimosa pudica*), which collapses and feigns death when disturbed, returning to normal once danger has passed. *In the same way that the release of our stress hormone cortisol catalyzes a reallocation of our energy from our vital organs to our arms and legs, thus enabling us to fight or flee from danger, plants have a chemical and biological response to stress that supports their survival.*

Responses can be mechanical, like the *Mimosa pudica* playing dead; they can be chemical, like the plant responding to the sound of caterpillars; and they can be electrical, as in the case of the Venus flycatcher. The flycatcher's electrical response is almost identical to nerve impulses in animals.

There are many examples of plant chemistry and behavior responding to environmental stimuli. And this happens not only in individual plants. Plants communicate threats to other plants in their species, sometimes causing all their kin in the neighborhood to change their biology en masse.

There are at least several ways plants have been shown to communicate with each other. *Impatiens* recognize their kin by a kind of communication transmitted among their roots. Acacia trees communicate via the air, producing tannin in response to threats like grazing. The scent of tannin becomes airborne and serves as a warning to neighboring acacia trees. These trees, in response, prepare for danger by producing tannin of their own. One threat to a single tree has now altered not only the tree's chemical composition, but also that of its neighbors.

Plants not only evolve and adapt to danger and threats, but to any circumstance. Evolutionary change depends on reproduction, and plants sometimes resort to quite complicated shenanigans to facilitate it. For example: one type of orchid secretes a smelly chemical that is identical to the one produced by a certain kind of bee. There is a certain kind of hornet that habitually feeds its young on this kind of bee, and so is frequently on the lookout for said bee. So, when the hornet smells the bee's scent emitting from the orchid, it pounces on the orchid, unwittingly serving as its pollinator. Unsatisfying for the hornet perhaps, but the clever orchid's goal is satisfied. Other clever orchids that lack nectar of their own tempt pollinators by secreting chemicals with the scents of flowers that actually deliver nectar.

All species conspire, consciously or otherwise, to survive and thrive, and their chemistry reflects this conspiracy. This applies within species but also to interspecies communication.

Interspecies relationships do not have to be antagonistic. For example, there is a certain fungus that lives harmoniously with leaf-cutting ants (*Atta sexdens rubropilosa*). The ants feed plant matter to the fungus, and should they happen to feed it a meal that is toxic to it, the fungus alerts the ants, that thereafter avoid feeding it that substance.

What does this all have to do with us? If we are indifferent or violent to plants, they may alter their qualities and actions—their very chemistry—in an attempt to protect themselves from us. This may initiate a chain reaction, altering kindred plants, other species, and the environment.

If we accept the theory of evolution, we have to believe that if we act in ways that plants perceive as threatening, they will unquestionably evolve to become, if not toxic to humans, at least inhospitable to us. Such an outcome would be inevitable, over time.

If plants change their qualities and actions, we cannot expect them to have the same effects that we have learned about in our schools and textbooks.

Charaka foresaw this, and he predicted that plant qualities would change over the four ages of time[8] in response to the changing conditions of those times. He taught that, in each age, as people's daily routines, diets, and thoughts suffered in quality, there would be a resulting one-quarter reduction in the "unctuousness, purity, tastes, potency, post-digestive effects, specific actions and qualities"[9] of plants. He wrote that this would be in inverse proportion to the increase of greed, attachment, avarice, malice, anger, worry, fear, and other ill-boding conditions. Considering that we are currently well into the fourth age, our plants—that is our food and medicine—are at least three-quarters less potent than their original nature.

The vicious cycle looks like this: we are indifferent to the sensibilities of plants and treat them disrespectfully. They evolve to become a little more toxic to us. Our bodies and intellects become a little weaker and a little more diseased. As our intellect becomes weaker, we are more likely to fall prey to ignoble qualities like excessive lust, anger, greed, attachment, and egoism, and therefore treat plants with more ignorant disregard. And round we go again, plants becoming less and less hospitable, and more and more toxic to us.

Along with human indifference, plants must also contend with polluted air, water, and earth, and seasonal disruptions due to climate change. How can the plants and herbs we are consuming as food and medicine be immune to all this? They can't and they aren't.

Charaka says that where seasons, rainfall, air, and earth become disturbed and polluted, "drugs lose their normal attributes and get impaired. Then there is impairment of the country because of the impairment of food and drinks."[10] These conditions breed epidemics, like cancer, diabetes, heart disease, and other lifestyle and environment-driven diseases.

With all this in mind, it seems prudent for us to pay closer attention to our relationships with plants: how to care for them, and how to grow, harvest, and prescribe them accordingly and judiciously.

If herb growers, harvesters, suppliers, physicians, and patients were to all to cooperate in a respectful process, perhaps our plants would be more potent and we would require fewer of them—and in smaller doses—to achieve equal or better results.

We stand at a unique time in evolution. We have made fantastic strides in modern technology. Concurrently, we have access to ancient wisdom in ancient medical texts, living individuals, communities—like those in the Amazon that, to date, have had minimal or zero contact with inhabitants of the so-called civilized world. These texts, individuals, and communities have recommended or nurtured and maintained respectful relationships with nature that have endured for millennia. Their knowledge of plants, healing, and how to cultivate sustainable relationships with our plants and planet is the product of thousands of years of observation and wisdom acquired from physical experimentation and Divine revelation.

It will be a pity if we cannot avail ourselves of their wisdom before we have poisoned our remedies. Modern CAM systems like Ayurveda are frequently hailed as being holistic and compassionate, but if we use Charaka's direction as a yardstick by which to measure our practices, we may find room for improvement.

43 Reflections on Part V

If we consider not only what effective medicine is for patients, but also what factors affect that medicine, we may well become more careful about how we grow, gather, procure, and prescribe plant medicines. We ourselves can have a medicinal or poisonous effect on the medicine we prescribe.

When we refine and purify our senses, our ability to diagnose and communicate with our patients improves. When we purify our senses, we purify ourselves. As we purify ourselves, our relationship with plants improves, and they may retain (or even regain) their potency. As it turns out, the very efforts we make at improving ourselves as human beings and physicians impact not only us and our patients, but plants and the planet as well.

PART VI

Compassion

Judge not, that ye be not judged.
For with what judgment ye judge, ye shall be judged.
And with what measure ye mete, it shall be measured to you again.
And why beholdest thou the mote that is in thy brother's eye,
but considerest not the beam that is in thine own eye?
MATTHEW 7: 1–3, THE BIBLE (KING JAMES VERSION)

When I began writing this book I didn't have a point to make. I didn't have a theme. I didn't have an agenda. I didn't have a take-home message. I was just up for exploring some practices and qualities central to the art of medicine.

We have considered the pursuit of knowledge through authority, perception, and inference. We have explored how to apply that knowledge to practical experience with patients, plants, and ourselves. We have explored the utility of an open mind and a rich toolbox in practicing dexterously, and the effect of good character on outcomes.

While sharing some of the ideas and practices that I have thought about frequently over the decades and over the course of writing this book, a few themes have emerged for me as most powerful.

I have become more convinced than ever that we—at least I—know very little. I have been struck again and again with how amazing it is that although we know very little, there are clearly happy side effects from the pursuit of knowledge alone, and from our efforts at becoming better physicians.

I am struck by the profound ramifications of refining our ability to deeply perceive our patients.

I am struck by how pursuit of knowledge, accumulation of experiences, efforts at practicing with an open mind and clear perception, all yield such a rich crop of healthy qualities central to the art of medicine: humility, confidence, healthy communication skills, empathy, increased dexterity, purity, and more accurate abilities to diagnose.

And I am struck by how, to the top of these qualities, rises one that may be most powerful: compassion. Compassion seems to be both a seed and a fruit. It seems to be a seed that, when nourished, yields deeper knowledge, richer experience, more dexterous medical intuition, and a purer heart. At the same time it also seems a natural fruit of cultivating these four qualities.

Compassion is the theme that most deeply emerges from my thoughts, reflections, and conversations with outstanding practitioners. If we can do nothing else—if we can't arrive at an elegant diagnosis, if we are at a loss for an effective treatment plan, if we are confused about our prescriptions—at least our patients will benefit from compassion. And, when we feel it for them, we are experiencing it ourselves.

Compassion is a lofty word. With almost patronizing undertones. Maybe this is why, while we often express how glad we are for someone's joy, we are not likely to respond to their sorrow by announcing how much compassion we feel for them. Compassion may not be something we feel *for* others. It may just be something we feel. It may not be something we aim in a certain direction, and bestow upon someone, but rather be more like a room or space we choose to enter. In this space, we can look for or focus on the Good, the Real, the Stable, the True inside ourselves, moment to moment, and attempt to perceive it in others. In fact, doing so may serve as a doorway into that compassionate space.

Refining our perceptive abilities, and practicing this with our patients and ourselves, as we have explored in this book, may itself be a practice in cultivating compassion. The more we are able to truly and clearly perceive our patients and ourselves, the less room there is for judgment in either case.

Judgment may well, in fact, be the opposite of compassion. When our senses are obstructed by ill will and judgment, we cloud our ability to perceive reality as it truly is. Perhaps this is why Charaka advises the physician, "You should not think ill of the patients even at the cost of your life."

Judgment differs from discernment. In discernment, we may conclude, for example, that someone's addiction is causing a disorder. This is an important part of doctoring. In judgment, however, we morally condemn the person for their addiction. This is not an important part of doctoring.

Judgment can have a pressing, strained, cold, and alienating effect on the spirit. When we sit in judgment of our patients, we lack mercy—it is as if we wish justice to be visited upon them. When we demand someone receive "just" punishment, we place ourselves squarely in the halls of justice. And if that is where we stand, we will have no choice but to be judged ourselves. Who among us would prefer justice to mercy when it comes to our own case?

There are times each of us may be desperate for mercy. In my own case, I would rather beg for mercy than fight for justice. Showing mercy to others is an extension of this sentiment.

I have failed at this more times than I can count. The impulse to judge others, in a myriad of small ways, is insidious, and the fight against it can be long, but in my experience, it is one worth fighting.

Avalokiteshvara Kuan-Yin is a Buddhist goddess and the archetype of compassion and mercy. Her name is variously translated as, "she who hears the sounds of the world," or "she who sees and hears the cries of the world," or "she who perceives the cries of suffering in the world."

If we strive to acquire knowledge, to purify our senses and our characters, to align with the Highest Good, and to accumulate experience and strategies, and if we are present to deeply listen to, see, and feel our patients, then we may find and cultivate compassion as well. And that may be the happiest side effect of all.

> *If you want others to be happy, practice compassion.*
> *If you want to be happy, practice compassion.*
> DALAI LAMA XIV, THE ART OF HAPPINESS

NOTES

Acknowledgments

1. "Raga, etc." includes *kama* (desire or lust), *krodha* (anger), *lobha* (greed), *mada* (arrogance), *matsarga* (jealousy), *dvesa* (hatred), *bhaya* (fear) and many such negative emotions.

2. *Ashtanga Hrdayam: Sutrasthanam*: I: 1, one of the three great, ancient Ayurvedic classic medical treatises.

Preface and Notes

1. 9369–286 BC, from *The Complete Works of Chuang Tzu.*

Introduction: The Art of Medicine and the Four Qualities of a Physician

1. *Sushruta Samhita: Sutrasthanam*: III: 47–52.

2. These four qualities are listed in *Charaka Samhita: Sutrasthanam*: IX: 6. (*śrute paryavadātatvam bahuśo dṛṣṭakarmatā | dākṣyaṃ śaucam iti jñeyaṃ vaidye guṇacatuṣṭayam ||*) The common translation of *paryavadāta-tvam* is "excellence in theoretical knowledge." A more accurate translation is "complete proficiency in what was taught," with medical knowledge being implied. I am using the more common translation for this book, as it is a bit more accessible and friendly and both translations lead us to question how, and from where, we learn what we learn and know what we know—the issues explored in Part I.

3. There are three main authoritative classical texts of Ayurvedic medicine. These three are the *brhat trayi* or, "Three Greats," and include *Charaka Samhita*, authored by Charaka, *Ashtanga Hrdayam*, authored by Vagbhata, and *Sushruta Samhita*, authored by Sushruta.

4. Physician, drug, attendant and patient, this is the quadruple which, if endowed with qualities, leads to alleviation of disorders (*Charaka Samhita: Sutrasthanam*: IX: 3).

5. *Charaka Samhita: Sutrasthanam*: IX: 10 and 24–25.

6. See footnote 2.

Part I: Excellence in Theoretical Knowledge

1. Ibid.

2. *Charaka Samhita: Sutrasthanam*: IX: 14–25.

3. These are the three most commonly listed forms of valid knowledge, and what I use in this book. There is a fourth that is sometimes listed: "knowledge based on rationale." While

Charaka doesn't include it in *Vimanasthanam*: IV: 1–4, he does in *Sutrasthana*: XI: 17. I don't include that in this book.

1. Authority: Questioning Our Sources of Knowledge

1. *Charaka Samhita: Vimanasthanam*: IV: 4.
2. *Sattva, rajas,* and *tamas* are considered to be three *mahagunas,* or archetypal qualities or states of being. Succinctly put, *sattva* could be defined as tranquil clarity, *rajas* as excessive activity, and *tamas* as inertia. In Ayurvedic classics, *sattva* is considered a pure state of mind, and *rajas* and *tamas* are considered qualities that pollute this pure state. The following definition of *sattva, rajas,* and *tamas,* from the *Bhagavad Gita,* is one I particularly like in the context of medicine: "That which in the beginning is like poison and whose semblance in transformation is nectar; that happiness, born from the tranquility of the spirit of oneself, is declared to be sattvic. That which in the beginning, through contact between the objects of the senses and the senses resembles nectar, and whose semblance in transformation is poison-like; that happiness is recorded as rajasic. That happiness which both in the beginning and in its consequence, deludes the self, arising from sleep, indolence and negligence, is declared to be tamasic" (*Bhagavad Gita*: XVIII: 37–39). And here is another: "That knowledge by which one sees one imperishable Being in all beings, undivided in the divided—know that knowledge to be *sattvic.* But that knowledge which sees all beings as separate entities, know that knowledge to be *rajasic.* That wherein one is irrationally and whimsically attached to a fragment of reality as if it were the whole, without knowledge of reality, *is tamasic*" (*Bhagavad Gita*: XVIII: 20–22).
3. *Charaka Samhita: Sutrasthanam*: XI: 18–19.
4. *Charaka Samhita: Vimanasthanam*: VIII: 3.
5. *Charaka Samhita: Vimanasthanam*: IV: 1–4.
6. Freedman, D. H. (2010) "Lies, damned lies, and medical science." *The Atlantic,* November.
7. Lehrer, J. (2010) "The truth wears off: is there something wrong with the scientific method?" *The New Yorker,* December 13.
8. Ioannidis, J. P. A. (2005) "Contradicted and initially stronger effects in highly cited clinical research." *JAMA 294*(2), 218–228.
9. Ioannidis, J. P. A. (2005) "Why most published research findings are false." *PLOS Medicine 2*(8), e124.
10. Lehrer, J. (2010) "The truth wears off: is there something wrong with the scientific method?" *The New Yorker,* December 13.
11. See www.ted.com/talks/ben_goldacre_what_doctors_don_t_know_about_the_drugs_they _prescribe.html
12. Freedman, D. H. (2010) "Lies, damned lies, and medical science." *The Atlantic,* November.
13. Ibid.
14. Kolata, G. (2013) "Scientific articles accepted (personal checks, too)." *New York Times,* April 7.
15. Ibid.
16. Lehrer, J. (2010) "The truth wears off: is there something wrong with the scientific method?" *The New Yorker,* December 13.
17. Nuzzo, R. (2014) "Scientific method: statistical errors P values, the "gold standard" of statistical validity, are not as reliable as many scientists assume." *Nature: International Weekly Journal of Science,* February 12.
18. Lehrer, J. (2010) "The truth wears off: is there something wrong with the scientific method?" *The New Yorker,* December 13.
19. Freedman, D. H. (2010) *"Lies, damned lies, and medical science." The Atlantic,* November.
20. Lehrer, J. (2010) "The truth wears off: is there something wrong with the scientific method?" *The New Yorker,* December 13.

21. Rehman, J. (2012) "Can the source of funding for medical research affect the results?" *Scientific American, September 23.* Available at http://blogs.scientificamerican.com/guest-blog/2012/09/23/can-the-source-of-funding-for-medical-research-affect-the-results

22. Ridker, P. M. and Torres, J. (2006) "Reported outcomes in major cardiovascular clinical trials funded by for-profit and not-for-profit organizations: 2000–2005." *JAMA 295*(19), 2270–2274.

23. For what can and cannot be patented, see www.legalmatch.com/law-library/article/what-cant-be-patented.html. For example, "You can patent pretty much anything under the sun that is made by man *except* laws of nature, physical phenomena, and abstract ideas. These categories are excluded subject matter from the scope of patents... Patent law classifies physical phenomena as products of nature. Thus, if your invention occurs in nature, it is a physical phenomenon and cannot be patented."

24. Grant, J. L., Ghosn, E. E., Axtell, R. C., Herges, K., Kuipers, H. F., Woodling, N. S., Andreasson, L. A., Herzenberg, L. A., Herzenberg, L. A. and Steinman, L. (2012) "Reversal of paralysis and reduced inflammation from peripheral administration of β-amyloid in TH1 and TH17 versions of experimental autoimmune encephalomyelitis." *Science Translational Medicine 4*(145), 145, August 1.

25. Writing Group for the Women's Health Initiative Investigators (2002) "Risks and benefits of estrogen plus progestin in healthy postmenopausal women: principal results from the Women's Health Initiative randomized controlled trial." *JAMA 288*(3), 321–333.

26. See www.ted.com/talks/ben_goldacre_what_doctors_don_t_know_about_the_drugs_they_prescribe.html

27. Angier, N. (2008) *The Canon: A Whirligig Tour of the Beautiful Basics.* Boston, MA and New York: Mariner Books, p.68.

28. O'Connor, A. (2014) "Advice from a vegan cardiologist." *New York Times*, August 6. Available at http://well.blogs.nytimes.com/2014/08/06/advice-from-a-vegan-cardiologist/?_php=true&_type=blogs&_r=0

2. Perception: Refining our Ability to Perceive Knowledge

1. *Charaka Samhita: Vimanasthanam*: IV: 1–4.

2. *Charaka Samhita: Sutrasthanam*: XI: 20.

3. *Charaka Samhita: Vimanasthanam*: IV: 5. This entire chapter is dedicated to the threefold sources of knowledge about disease characteristics.

4. Ramachandran, V. S. and Blakeslee, S. (1998) *Phantoms in the Brain: Probing the Mysteries of the Human Mind.* New York: William Morrow and Company, Inc., p.xiii.

5. Diaz, M. and Neuhauser, D. (2005) "Pasteur and parachutes: when statistical process control is better than a randomized controlled trial." *Quality & Safety in Health Care 14*, 140–143.

6. Smith, G. C. S. and Pell, J. P. (2003) "Parachute use to prevent death and major trauma related to gravitational challenge: systematic review of randomized controlled trials." *British Medical Journal 327*(7429), 1459–1461.

7. Bartlett, R. H., Roloff, D. W., Cornell, R. G., French Andrews, A., Dillon, P. W. and Zwischenberger, J. B. (1985) "Extracorporeal circulation in neonatal respiratory failure: a prospective randomized study." *Pediatrics 76*(4), 479–487, October 1.

8. "Quick, inexpensive and a 90 percent cure rate." Available at www.mayoclinic.org/medical-professionals/clinical-updates/digestive-diseases/quick-inexpensive-90-percent-cure-rate

9. Bechara, A., Damásio, A. R., Damásio, H., Anderson, S. W. (1994) "Insensitivity to future consequences following damage to human prefrontal cortex." *Cognition 50*(1–3), 7–15.

10. Interview with Dr. Eduardo Cardona-Sanclemente: "First, You Have To Be" by Richard Whittaker, October 22, 2014. See more at www.conversations.org/story.php?sid=407#sthash.yHGJp9i7.dpuf

11. Montague, E., Chen, P., Xu, J., Chewning, B. and Barrett, B. (2013) "Nonverbal interpersonal interactions in clinical encounters and patient perceptions of empathy." *Journal of Participatory Medicine,* 5: e33, August 14.

12. Interview with Dr. Eduardo Cardona-Sanclemente: "First, You Have To Be" by Richard Whittaker, October 22, 2014. See more at www.conversations.org/story.php?sid=407#sthash.yHGJp9i7.dpuf

13. Sant Ajaib Singh ji Maharaj (2007) *In Search of the Gracious One: An Account in His Own Words of the Spiritual Search and Discipleship of Sant Ajaib Singh* (compiled by Michael Mayo-Smith). Manchester, NH: Keystone Press, p.210.

14. Blakemore, C. and Cooper, G. F. (1970) "Development of the brain depends on the visual environment." *Nature 228,* 447–448.

15. See www.forteantimes.com/strangedays/science/20/questioning_perceptual_blindness.html

16. Vedantam, S. (2005) "Social network's healing power is borne out in poorer nations." *Washington Post,* June 27, A01.

17. Sacks, O. (2010) *The Mind's Eye.* New York and Toronto: Alfred A. Knopf, p.204.

18. Ibid, p.205 (footnote 1).

19. Ibid, pp.208–211.

20. Ibid, p.233.

21. Ibid, p.219.

22. Doidge, N. (2007) *The Brain that Changes Itself: Stories of Personal Triumph from the Frontiers of Brain Science.* London: Penguin Books, p.304.

23. Ibid, p.289.

24. See http://blogs.artinfo.com/lacmonfire/tag/getty-kouros

25. See www.getty.edu/art/gettyguide/artObjectDetails?artobj=12908

26. Murphymay, K. (2014) "Psst. Look over here." *New York Times,* May 16. *Available at www.nytimes.com/2014/05/17/sunday-review/the-eyes-have-it.html*

27. Montague, E., Chen, P., Xu, J., Chewning, B. and Barrett, B. (2013) "Nonverbal interpersonal interactions in clinical encounters and patient perceptions of empathy." *Journal of Participatory Medicine,* 5:e33, August 14.

28. Murphymay, K. (2014) "Psst. Look over here." *New York Times,* May 16. *Available at www.nytimes.com/2014/05/17/sunday-review/the-eyes-have-it.html*

29. Pönkänen, L. M., Alhoniemi, A., Leppänen, J. M. and Hietanen, J. K. (2011) "Does it make a difference if I have an eye contact with you or with your picture?" *Social Cognitive and Affective Neuroscience 6*(4), 486–494.

30. Montague, E., Chen, P., Xu, J., Chewning, B. and Barrett, B. (2013) "Nonverbal interpersonal interactions in clinical encounters and patient perceptions of empathy." *Journal of Participatory Medicine,* 5:e33, August 14.

31. Finkel, M. (2014) "The strange & curious tale of the last true hermit." *Golf Digest,* September. Available at www.gq.com/news-politics/newsmakers/201409/the-last-true-hermit

32. Singh, K. (1960) *Naam or Word: In the Beginning Was the Word…* San Jose, CA: Ruhani Satsang Books, pp.43–45.

33. This is how Kirpal Singh describes the four types of communication, using the transliteration, "baikhri," "madhma," pashianti," and "para." Other teachers teach and transliterate these four categories in other ways. One variation, for example, is that the four seats are: "vaikari" in the throat, "madhyma" (or madhyama) in the heart, "pashyanti" in the navel, and "para" in the muladhara chakra, or near the perineum. I find it hard to communicate from the perineum and so, because of that, and because Kirpal Singh is a prominent teacher in my lineage, I am presenting his perspective here, but using more current and common transliteration of the terms.

34. "The incredible story of how leopard Diabolo became Spirit—Anna Breytenbach, 'animal communicator,'" a 13-minute video clip that went viral: www.youtube.com/watch?v=gvwHHMEDdT0

35. From Anna Breytenbach's email newsletter, received on April, 30, 2014. You can subscribe to this newsletter at www.animalspirit.org

36. For a more complete description and guided visualization, listen to the Prana CD found at http://drclaudiawelch.com/shop/cds, with emphasis on the "Dissolving Obstructions" track.

37. There are also the *vignanamayakosha* and the *anandamayakosha*, but these are not relevant to this context.

38. Montague, E., Chen, P., Xu, J., Chewning, B. and Barrett, B. (2013) "Nonverbal interpersonal interactions in clinical encounters and patient perceptions of empathy." *Journal of Participatory Medicine*, 5:e33, August 14.

39. *Bhagavad Gita*: II: 66.

40. Sacks, O. (2010) *The Mind's Eye*. New York and Toronto: Alfred A. Knopf, final chapter.

41. Tongue J. R., Epps, H. R. and Forese, L. L. (2005) "Communication skills for patient-centered care: research-based, easily learned techniques for medical interviews that benefit orthopaedic surgeons and their patients." *Journal of Bone and Joint Surgery* 87, 652–658.

42. Cousins, N. (1985) "How patients appraise physicians." *The New England Journal of Medicine* 313(22), 1422.

43. Del Canale, S., Louis, D. Z., Maio, V., Wang, X., Rossi, G., Hojat, M. and Gonnella, J. S. (2012) "The relationship between physician empathy and disease complications: an empirical study of primary care physicians and their diabetic patients in Parma, Italy." *Academic Medicine* 87(9), 1243–1249, September.

3. Inference: The Role of Prediction in Knowledge

1. *Charaka Samhita: Sutrasthanam*: XI: 21–22.

2. Grant, J. L., Ghosn, E. E., Axtell, R. C., Herges, K., Kuipers, H. F., Woodling, N. S., Andreasson, L. A., Herzenberg, L. A., Herzenberg, L. A. and Steinman, L. (2012) "Reversal of paralysis and reduced inflammation from peripheral administration of β-amyloid in TH1 and TH17 versions of experimental autoimmune encephalomyelitis." *Science Translational Medicine 4*(145), 145, August 1; Kurnellas, M. P., Adams, C. M., Sobel, R. A., Steinman, L. and Rothbard, J. B. (2013) "Amyloid fibrils composed of hexameric peptides attenuate neuroinflammation." *Science Translational Medicine 5*, 179ra42; Hohlfeld, R. and Wekerle, H. (2012) "β-amyloid: enemy or remedy?" *Science Translational Medicine 4*, 145fs24.

3. A good little interview that describes this is at www.sciencefriday.com/segment/04/05/2013/amyloid-proteins-help-paralyzed-mice-walk-again.html

4. Ornish, D., Magbanua, M. J. M., Weidner, G., Weinberg, V., Kemp, C., Green, C., Mattie, M. D., Marlin, R., Simko, J., Shinohara, K., Hagg, C. M. and Carroll, P. R. (2008) "Changes in prostate gene expression in men undergoing an intensive nutrition and lifestyle intervention." *Proceedings of the National Academy of Sciences 105*(24), 8369–8374, June 17. Available at www.ncbi.nlm.nih.gov/pmc/articles/PMC2430265/

4. Reflections on Part I

1. *Charaka Samhita: Vimanasthanam*: IV: 12.

2. Montague, E., Chen, P., Xu, J., Chewning, B. and Barrett, B. (2013) "Nonverbal interpersonal interactions in clinical encounters and patient perceptions of empathy." *Journal of Participatory Medicine*, 5:e33, August 14.

Part II: Extensive Practical Experience: Things We May Not Learn in School

1.   *Charaka Samhita: Sutrasthanam*: IX: 21–23.

7. Doctor as Educator

1.   Svoboda, R. E. (1988) *Prakriti: Your Ayurvedic Constitution*. Albuquerque, NM: Geocom, Limited, p.2.

2.   Crow, D. (2000) *In Search of the Medicine Buddha: A Himalayan Journey*. New York: Tarcher/ Putnam Penguin. Quote attributed to Dr. Ngawang Chopel, p.310.

8. Treat Complicated with Simple

1.   Campbell, T. C. and Campbell, T. M. (2006) *The China Study: The Most Comprehensive Study of Nutrition Ever Conducted and the Startling Implications for Diet, Weight Loss and Long-term Health*. Dallas, TX: BenBella Books, Inc., p.238.

10. Patients Should Get Better

1.   *Sadhya* diseases are curable. This category is further divided into two categories: *sukhasadhya*— or diseases that are easily curable within a short amount of time; and *kruchchhasadhya*—diseases that are curable with difficulty. *Asadhya* diseases, as the name suggests, are the opposite of *sadhya*. They are incurable. *Asadhya* is also divided into two categories: *yapya*—illnesses that, while incurable, can be managed with remedies or treatments; and *anukarma*—incurable illnesses that are also unmanageable with remedies or treatments.

2.   Buechner, F. (2014) Blog, August 11. Available at www.frederickbuechner.com/content/ story, originally published in Buechner, F. (2009) *Whistling in the Dark: A Doubter's Dictionary*. New York: HarperCollins e-books.

12. Healing Through Environment, Co-Workers, and Protocols (This is Not as Boring as It Sounds)

1.   See www.sun-tes.ru

2.   Interview with Shen Yun Symphony Orchestra composer, Gao Yuan. Available at www. shenyun.com/whatsnew/article/e/QrYhYohmjxM/composer-interview-gao-yuan.html

3.   Ackerman, J. M., Nocera, C. C. and Bargh, J. A. (2010) "Incidental haptic sensations influence social judgments and decisions." *Science 328*(5986), 1712–1715, June 25.

4.   Schneider, I. K., Rutjens, B. T., Jostmann, N. B. and Lakens, D. (2011) "Weighty matters: importance literally feels heavy." *Social Psychological and Personality Science 2*, pp.474–478, September 1.

5.   Zhong, C.-B. and Leonardelli, G. J. (2008) "Cold and lonely: does social exclusion literally feel cold?" *Psychological Science 19*, 838–842, September.

6.   Williams, L. E. and Bargh, J. A. (2008) "*Experiencing physical warmth promotes interpersonal warmth.*" *Science 322*(5901), 606–607, October 24.

16. The Role of Story in Diagnosis, Treatment, and Compliance

1. Stewart, M., Brown, J. B., Donner, A., McWhinney, I. R., Oates, J., Weston, W. W. and Jordan, J. J. (2000) "The impact of patient-centered care on outcomes." *Family Practice 49*(9), 796–804, September.

2. Fong Ha, J. and Longnecker, N. (2010) "Doctor-patient commumication: a review." *The Ochsner Journal 10*(1), 38–43, Spring. Available at www.ncbi.nlm.nih.gov/pmc/articles/PMC3096184/

3. Platt, F. W. and Keating, K. N. (2007) "Differences in physician and patient perceptions of uncomplicated UTI symptom severity: understanding the communication gap." *International Journal of Clinical Practice 61*(2), 303–308, February.

17. Confidence vs. Cockiness

1. Dossey, L. D. (1993) *Healing Words*. New York: HarperCollins Publishers, chapter 8.

2. Toone, W. M. (1973) "Effects of Vitamin E: good and bad." *New England Journal of Medicine 289*, 689–698.

3. Anderson, T. W. (1974) "Vitamin E in angina pectoris." *Canadian Medical Association Journal 110*, 401–406; Gillian, R., Mondell, B. and Warbasse, J. R. (1977) "Quantitative evaluation of Vitamin E in the treatment of angina pectoris." *American Heart Journal 93*, 444–449.

4. Uhlenhuth, E. H., Cantor, A., Neustadt, J. O. and H. E. Payson (1959) "The symptomatic relief of anxiety with meprobamate, phenobarbital and placebo." *American Journal of Psychiatry 115*, 905–910.

5. Solfvin, J. (1984) "Mental Healing." In S. Krippner (ed.) *Advances in Parapsychological Research, Volume 4* (pp.55–56). Jefferson, NC: McFarland and Company. See also: Engelhardt, D. M. and Margolis, R. (1967) "Drug Identity, Doctor Conviction and Outcome." In H. Brill (ed.) *Proceedings of the Fifth International Congress of Neuropsychopharmacology*. Amsterdam: Excerpta Medica Foundation; Feldman, P. E. (1956) "The personal element in psychiatric research." *American Journal of Psychiatry 113*, 52–54; Joyce, C. R. B. (1962) "Differnces between physicians as revealed by clinical trials." *Proceedings of the Toyal Society of Medicine 55*, 776; Modell, W. and Houde, R. W. (1958) "Factors influencing the clinical evaluation of drugs: with special reference to the double-blind technique." *Journal of the American Medical Association 167*, 2190–2199; Williams, M. and McGee, T. F. (1962) "The bias of the drug administration in judgments of the effects of psychopharmacological agents." *Journal of Nervous and Mental Disease 135*, 569–573.

19. Cake or Death? Choosing Hope

1. Levinson, W., Gorawara-Bhat, R. and Lamb, J. (2000) "A study of patient clues and physician responses in primary care and surgical settings." *JAMA 284*(8), 1021–1027.

2. Peterson C. *et al.* (1993) "Optimism and bypass surgery." In C. Peterson, S. F. Maier and M. E. P. Seligman (eds) *Learned Helplessness: A Theory for the Age of Personal Control*. New York: Oxford University Press.

3. Weiss, R. B., Woolf, S. H., Demakos, E., Holland, J. F., Berry, D. A., Falkson, G., Cirrincione, C. T., Robbins, A., Bothun, S., Henderson, I. C. and Norton, L. (2003) "Natural history of more than 20 years of node-positive primary breast carcinoma treated with cyclophosphamide, methotrexate, and fluorouracil-based adjuvant chemotherapy: a study by the Cancer and Leukemia Group." *Journal of Clinical Oncology*, 1825–1835, May 1.

20. Sexual Abuse

1. According to the U.S. Department of Justice's National Crime Victimization Survey (NCVS), there are an average of 293,066 victims (age 12 or older) of rape and sexual assault in the US each year. Since there are 525,600 minutes in a non-leap year, there are 31,536,000 seconds per year. When we divide this by 293,066, this means that there is one sexual assault every 107 seconds.

2. Tjaden, P. and Thoennes, N. (1998) *Prevalence, Incidence and Consequences of Violence Against Women: Findings from the National Violence Against Women Survey.* Washington, DC: National Institute of Justice Centers for Disease Control and Prevention. Available at www.ncjrs.gov/pdffiles/172837.pdf

21. Addictions

1. *Charaka Samhita: Sutrasthanam:* VII: 36–38.

2. Esser, M.B., Hedden, S. L., Kanny, D., Brewer, R. D., Gfroerer, J. C. and Naimi, T. S. (2014) "Prevalence of alcohol dependence among US adult drinkers, 2009–2011." *Preventing Chronic Disease 11,* 140329.

3. Ibid.

4. Ibid.

5. Ibid.

6. Ibid.

7. Ibid.

8. Ibid.

9. NIH (National Institute on Alcohol Abuse and Alcoholism) (2005) *Helping Patients Who Drink Too Much: A Clinician's Guide.* NIH Pub. No. 05–3769. Bethesda, MD: NIH. Available at http://pubs.niaaa.nih.gov/publications/AA66/AA66.htm

10. See www.heroesinrecovery.com/about

11. This section is highly influenced by conversations between the author and Durga Leela, B.A., founder of Yoga of Recovery, on May 20, 2014.

12. Lawford, C. K. (2010) *Moments of Clarity: Voices from the Front Lines of Addiction and Recovery.* New York: William Morrow Paperbacks.

13. Doidge, N. (2007) *The Brain that Changes Itself: Stories of Personal Triumph from the Frontiers of Brain Science.* London: Penguin Books, p.204.

14. Mager, D. (2014) "What constitutes a spiritual awakening? Awakenings of the spirit come in many different shapes and sizes." *Psychology Today,* April 14.

15. Rick Silberman, Facebook post to the author on Wednesday, November 5, 2014.

16. Information and statistics in this section are from NIH (National Institute on Alcohol Abuse and Alcoholism) (2005) *Helping Patients Who Drink Too Much: A Clinician's Guide.* NIH Pub. No. 05–3769. Bethesda, MD: NIH. Available at http://pubs.niaaa.nih.gov/publications/AA66/AA66.htm

17. Noble, E. P. (2000) *"Addiction may be in the genes." Los Angeles Times,* December 4.

22. Mental Illness

1. Education: University of Ouagadougou, B.A.s in Sociology, Literature, and Linguistics, 1981; M.A. in World Literature, 1982; Sorbonne, University of Paris, D.E.A. in Political Science, 1983; Brandeis University, M.A., 1984; Ph.D. in Literature, 1990.

2. Marohn, S. (2003) *The Natural Medicine Guide to Schizophrenia.* Charlottesville, VA: Hampton Roads Publishing Company, Inc., pp.178–179 (featuring Malidoma Patrice Somé).

3. Ibid.
4. Ibid.
5. CDC (Centers for Disease Control and Prevention) "Preventing suicide." Available at www.
    cdc.gov/features/preventingsuicide
6. Ibid.
7. Finkelstein, B. (2013) "Perfect Moments." The Moth podcast, September 2. Available at
    http://themoth.org/posts/storytellers/brian-finkelstein

23. Eating Disorders

1. For more information about *abhyanga*, see http://drclaudiawelch.com/resources/articles/
    abhyanga-ayurvedic-oil-massage/

25. Determining the Severity of a Crisis

1. *Charaka Samhita: Vimanasthanam*: VII: 3.
2. Singh, S. (2007) *Spiritual Gems*. Punjab, India: Radha Soami Satsang Beas, p.163.

Part III: Dexterity: The Value of Flexible Medicine

1. *Charaka Samhita: Vimanasthanam*: VIII: 15.
2. Fred assures us that "dexterity," is indeed a good translation of the sanskrit word Charaka
    uses—*dakshya*. It relates to the dexterity of the right hand—usually people's dominant hand.
    Email correspondence with Fred Smith, from June 8, 2012: "The word dākṣya is related
    etymologically to the English "dexterity," the primary Sanskrit word being dakṣa (dākṣya
    is derived from this). This meaning extends to its derivative dakṣiṇā, which means "south,"
    hence "right" as in right side or right hand. The primary direction in India was the east. Thus
    south was at the right as you faced east. Thus south and right hand are the same word. It's the
    dextrous side, assuming the predominance of right-handedness. Hence dakṣiṇā, gift to priests,
    etc., are rewards for their priestly dexterity."

28. Reaching Beyond Our Own Field

1. *Sushruta Samhita: Sutrasthanam*: IV: 5–6.

29. When the Front Door Is Locked, Use the Back Door, or Even a Window

1. *Huang di Nei Jing*, Chapter 11: Further Discourse on the Five Zang Viscera.

31. Loopholes: Thinking Outside the Box

1. *Charaka Samhita: Sarirasthanam*: IV: 13.

Part IV: Purity: Are We Medicine or Poison?

1. *Charaka Samhita: Sutrasthanam*: IX: 20.

2. *Charaka Samhita: Sutrasthanam*: IX: 26.

3. *Charaka Samhita: Vimanasthanam*: VIII: 8.

4. *Charaka Samhita: Vimanasthanam*: VIII: part of 13.

5. *Sushruta Samhita: Sutrasthanam*: X: 2.

33. Spiritual Powers vs. Effect of Character

1. Kaplan, S. H., Greenfield, S. and Ware, J. E. (1989) "Assessing the effects of physician-patient interactions on the outcomes of chronic disease." *Medical Care 27*(3 Suppl.), S110–S127, March.

2. Dinacharya chapter in *Charaka Samhita: Sushruta Samhita*: VIII: 29.

3. Rehman, S. U., Nietert, P. J., Cope, D. W. and Kilpatrick, A. O. (2005) "What to wear today? Effect of doctor's attire on the trust and confidence of patients." *The American Journal of Medicine 118*(11), 1279–1286, November.

4. Interview with Dr. Eduardo Cardona-Sanclemente: "First, You Have To Be" by Richard Whittaker, October 22, 2014. See more at www.conversations.org/story.php?sid=407#sthash. yHGJp9i7.dpuf

5. Little, P., Everitt, H., Williamson, I., Warner, G., Moore, M., Gould, C., Ferrier, K. and Payne, S. (2001) "Observational study of effect of patient centredness and positive approach on outcomes of general practice consultations." *British Medical Journal 323*(7318), 908–911, October 20.

6. Kaplan, S. H., Greenfield, S. and Ware, J. E. (1989) "Assessing the effects of physician-patient interactions on the outcomes of chronic disease." *Medical Care 27*(3 Suppl.), S110–S127, March.

7. Sant Ajaib Singh ji Maharaj (2007) *In Search of the Gracious One: An Account in His Own Words of the Spiritual Search and Discipleship of Sant Ajaib Singh* (compiled by Michael Mayo-Smith). Manchester, NH: Keystone Press, p.211.

8. Mascaro, J. S., Rilling, J. K., Negi, L. T. and Raison, C. L. (2013) "Compassion meditation enhances empathic accuracy and related neural activity." *Social Cognitive and Affective Neuroscience 8*(1), 48–55, January.

9. Sant Ajaib Singh ji Maharaj (2007) *In Search of the Gracious One: An Account in His Own Words of the Spiritual Search and Discipleship of Sant Ajaib Singh* (compiled by Michael Mayo-Smith). Manchester, NH: Keystone Press, p.209.

10. Sant Ajaib Singh ji Maharaj (2007) *In Search of the Gracious One: An Account in His Own Words of the Spiritual Search and Discipleship of Sant Ajaib Singh* (compiled by Michael Mayo-Smith). Manchester, NH: Keystone Press, p.210.

11. Sant Ajaib Singh ji Maharaj 2007, p.211.

12. Larre, C. and Rochat de la Vallee, E. (1990) "The practitioner-patient relationship: wisdom from the Chinese classics. Notes from a seminar." *Journal of Traditional Acupuncture 91*, 14–50, Winter.

34. The Mechanics of Emotional Contagion: Who Affects Whom?

1. Ramachandran, V. (2009) "The neurons that shaped civilization." TEDIndia 2009, 7:43, filmed November. Available at www.ted.com/talks/vs_ramachandran_the_neurons_that_shaped_civilization#t-130602

2. Ibid.

3. Larre, C. and Rochat de la Vallee, E. (1990) "The practitioner-patient relationship: wisdom from the Chinese classics. Notes from a seminar." *Journal of Traditional Acupuncture 91*, 14–50, Winter, p.48.

4. Zak, P. (2011) "Trust, morality—and oxytocin?" TEDGlobal 2011, 16:34, filmed July. Available at www.ted.com/talks/paul_zak_trust_morality_and_oxytocin?awesm=on.ted.com_Zak&utm_campaign=&utm_medium=on.ted.com-static&utm_source=echoparenting.org&utm_content=awesm-publisher

35. Supporting Change Through Appropriate Familiarity, Love, and Focus

1. Martin *et al.*, Reducing Social Stress Elicits Emotional Contagion of Pain in Mouse and Human Strangers, Current Biology (2015), published online Jan. 15, 2015. http://dx.doi.org/10.1016/j.cub.2014.11.028

2. See www.mcgill.ca/medicine/channels/news/secret-empathy-241112

36. Good Company

1. *Charaka Samhita: Vimanasthanam*: VIII: 15.

2. *Charaka Samhita: Vimanasthanam*: VIII: 14.

Part V: The Four Qualities of Effective Medicine

1. *Charaka Samhita: Sutrasthanam*: IX: 7.

2. *Charaka Samhita: Kalpasthanam*: I: 10–11. Sushruta says that the gatherer should look towards the north at the time of harvesting, and that plants should be regarded as partaking in the virtues of the ground they grow on. *Sushruta Samhita: Sutrasthanam*: XXXVII: 2. Other than these passages, I have not found other passages in the *brhat trayi* that relate to the attitude one should cultivate while harvesting. This may be because it was taken as a given that practitioners would treat plants this way. Just as it is unnecessary to counsel practitioners not to hit their patients, it may have been assumed that practitioners would consider the wellbeing of the plant medicine on which they depended.

3. *Charaka Samhita: Sutrasthanam*: I: 120–123.

4. *Charaka Samhita: Sutrasthanam*: IX: 7.

39. Abundance

1. Ramabhadran Pillai, R. (2002) "Ayurvedic medicine exporters in a fix." *The Hindu*, Sunday, January 27. Available at www.thehindu.com/2002/01/27/stories/2002012703210300.htm. The Commerce Ministry's notification No. 2 (RE-98/1997-2002).

40. Suitability

1. Good memory, obedience, fearlessness, and uninhibited expression—these are the four qualities of a patient. *Charaka Samhita: Sutrasthanam*: IX: 9.
2. *Charaka Samhita: Sutrasthanam*: XXVI: 12.
3. Author of *Ashtanga Hrdayam*, a fundamental Ayurvedic text.
4. Gogte, vaidya v.m. (trans.) (2000) *Dravyagunavignyana*: I: 35. S. Ramakrishnan (ed.). Mumbai: Bharatiya vidya bhavan.

41. Multiple Form

1. See www.theplantlist.org/1.1/statistics
2. Quoted in Mehl-Madrona, L. (2007) *Narrative Medicine: The Use of History and Story in the Healing Process*. Rochester, VT: Bear & Company. In endnote #4 for Chapter 3: Tom Lovejoy (1996) "How much is an elephant worth?" *Nature 382*, 594. I was not able to find this original source.
3. Taylor, L. (2004) *The Healing Power of Rainforest Herbs: A Guide to Understanding and Using Herbal Medicinals*. New Hyde Park, NY: Square One Publishers, Chapter 2.
4. Plotkin, M. J. (1994) *Tales of a Shaman's Apprentice: An Ethnobotanist Searches for New Medicines in the Amazon Rain Forest*. Hawthorn, VIC: Penguin Books Australia, p.13.
5. "Measuring the daily destruction of the world's rainforests." *Scientific American,* November 19, 2009. Available at www.scientificamerican.com/article/earth-talks-daily-destruction/
6. Plotkin, M. J. (1993) *Tales of a Shaman's Apprentice: An Ethnobotanist Searches for New Medicines in the Amazon Rain Forest*. Hawthorn, VIC: Penguin Books Australia, p.13.
7. "Can a plant be altruistic?" *ScienceDaily*, November 12, 2009. Available at www.sciencedaily. com/releases/2009/11/091111092047.htm

42. Potency

1. *Charaka Samhita: Sutrasthanam*: XXVI: 13.
2. *Charaka Samhita: Vimanasthanam*: III: 4–8.
3. Geddes, P. (1920) *The Life and Work of Sir Jagadis C. Bose*. New York: Longmans, p.146.
4. Backster, C. (1968) "Evidence of a primary perception in plant life." *International Journal of Parapsychology X*(4), 329–349, Winter.
5. Koechlin, F. (2009) "The dignity of plants." *Plant Signaling & Behavior 4*(1), 78–79, January.
6. Karpiński, S. and Szechyńska-Hebda, M. (2010) "Secret life of plants: from memory to intelligence." *Landes Bioscience 5*(11), November 1.
7. Appel, H. M. and Cocroft, R. B. (2014) "*Plants respond to leaf vibrations caused by insect herbivore chewing.*" *Oecologica 175*, 1257–1266. Available at http://link.springer.com/article/10.1007%2Fs00442-014-2995-6#page-1.
8. Satya Yuga, the Age of Truth, the golden age of mankind. After Satya Yuga come three, progressively more morally poor and physically weaker ages: Treta Yuga or Silver Age, Dvapara Yuga or Bronze Age, and the present yuga, Kali Yuga, or the Iron Age.
9. In the beginning of the Satya Yuga, because of the noble mind, qualities and actions of the people, the earth, etc. got endowed with all the good qualities, as a result of which excellent tastes, potencies, *vipaka* and specific actions were manifested in food grains.

    At the end of the Satya Yuga, some rich people got heaviness in their bodies due to over-indulgence. They suffered from fatigue because of the heaviness of the body. Fatigue gave rise to laziness; laziness caused them to accumulate things; accumulation let to the attachment for these things; and attachment resulted in greed.

During Treta Yuga, greed gave rise to malice; malice gave rise to false statements; and from false statements arose passion, anger, vanity, dislikes, cruelty, infliction of injury, fear, sorrow, grief, worry, anxiety, etc. Therefore, during Treta Yuga, a quarter of *dharma* disappeared. Because of this, the life span of human beings was reduced by a quarter. Similarly, there was reduction in the attributes of earth, etc., by one quarter. Because of the reduction of these attributes, there was diminution by one quarter of the unctuousness, purity, tastes, potency, *vipakas*, specific actions and qualities of grains.

Because of the reduction by a quarter of the attributes of diets and regimens, there was an unusual change in the maintenance of equilibrium of tissue elements, and there was vitiation of *agni* and *maruta* by which, first of all, bodies of living beings got afflicted with diseases, vis. *jvara*, etc. Therefore the lifespan of living beings underwent gradual diminution. (24)

Thus it is said, *dharma* and qualities of living beings got reduced in quarters gradually by the passage of each *yuga*... (25) (*Charaka Samhita: Vimanasthanam*: III: 24–25)

10.   *Charaka Samhita: Vimanasthanam*: III: 19–20.

INDEX